dance
your way to
fitness

Natalie Blenford

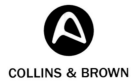

COLLINS & BROWN

First published in Great Britain in 2007 by
Collins & Brown
151 Freston Road
London
W10 6TH

An imprint of Anova Books Company Ltd

Distributed in the United States and Canada by
Sterling Publishing Co, 387 Park Avenue South, New
York, NY 10016, USA.

1 3 5 7 9 8 6 4 2 1

British Library Cataloguing-in-Publication Data:
A catalogue record for this book is available from the
British Library.

ISBN 1 84340 388 9

Commissioning Editor: Victoria Alers-Hankey
Editors: Chris Stone and Fiona Corbridge
Design Manager: Gemma Wilson
Design: Jo Knowles
Photographs: Janie Airey
Models: Satu Suominen, Caroline Graham, Jennifer
Tanarez

Reproduction by Anorax Imaging Ltd
Printed and bound by SNP Leefung
Printers Ltd, China

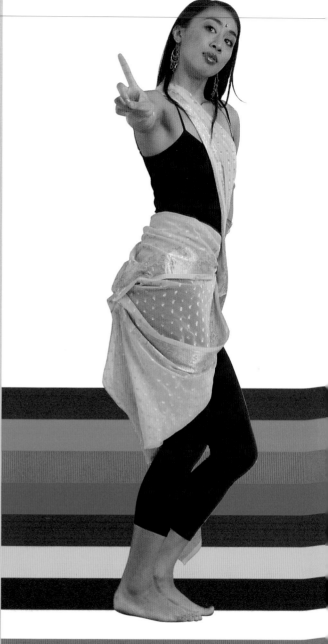

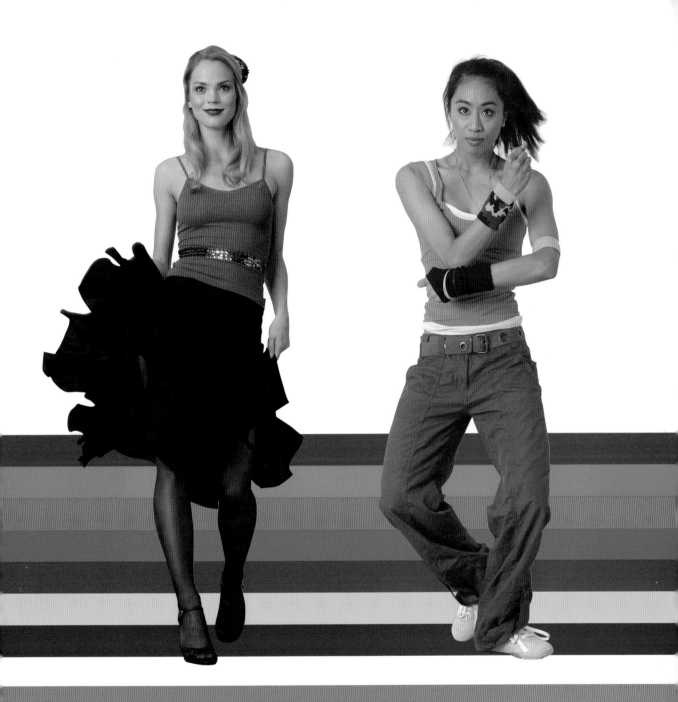

Contents

Introduction
1. Getting Started   4
2. The Warm Up   20
3. The Hip Hop Workout   36
4. The Broadway Workout   58
5. The Latin Workout   80
6. The Bollywood Workout   98
7. The Burlesque Workout   120
Index   141

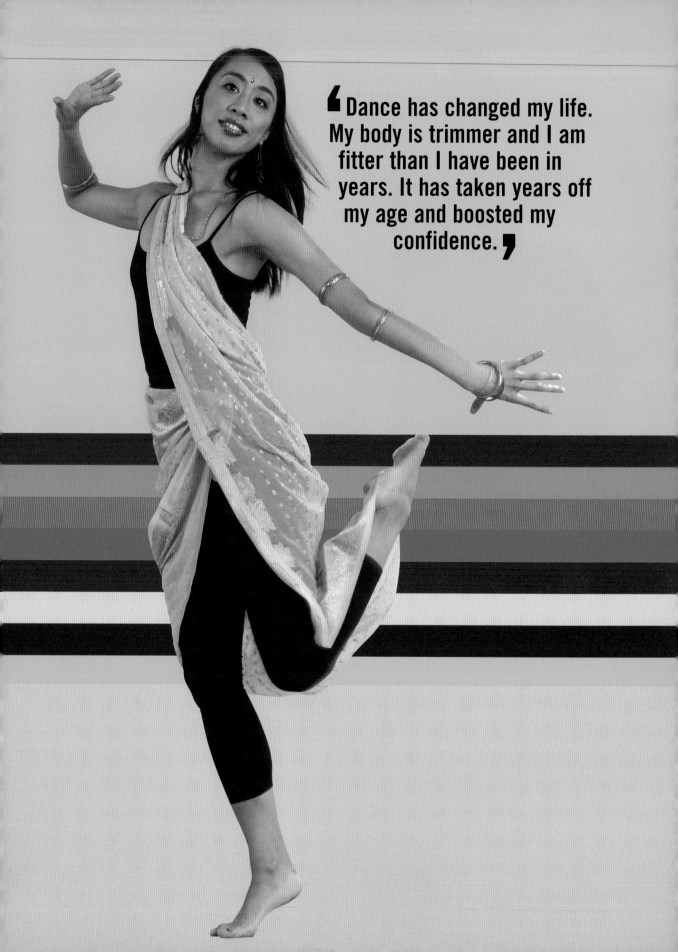

"Dance has changed my life. My body is trimmer and I am fitter than I have been in years. It has taken years off my age and boosted my confidence. "

Introduction

Dance is so much fun – it doesn't instantly seem like fitness but you only have to look at the bodies of J-Lo and Beyonce to know that dancing is one of Hollywood's favourite ways to get fit and fabulous fast. In fact, dancing has never been more fashionable – leggings, leg warmers and leotards have been fighting their way onto the shelves of sports stores bringing fun and femininity to fit kit and funky dance classes from hip hop to disco have found their place on gym timetables.

But this isn't just a fad, dance's fitness credentials are entirely serious – it really is a great way to shape up – combining fat blasting cardio, with top-to-toe toning. And what's more, it's great fun and can be practised anywhere. You don't need expensive equipment or complicated props to get started. You just need a small space, a CD of music you love and a willingness to push yourself outside of your usual exercise comfort zone. If you've never danced before in your life, don't fret. The workouts in this book are just as suitable for beginners as they are for seasoned dancers. And if you can't remember the last time you actually put your gym-kit on and did any exercise, this book really is perfect for you! The workouts can be danced at any pace, so if you're new to exercise and want to take things slowly, choose a track from the 'Getting Fit' play list and dance to a slow tempo until you feel yourself getting stronger and fitter. Then you can move on to a track from the 'Fighting Fit' play list, before progressing to fast tracks from the 'Super Fit' playlist when you really are super-fit.

❜ ...you're sure to have a great time! ❜

This book might not turn you into a professional dancer overnight, but use it three times per week for a month and you will soon notice positive changes all over your body. Most of all, like the case studies in this book, you'll find your confidence will soar as you connect with your sexy new body.

Because dancing is as individual as you are, we've covered five fun dance styles and a quiz to help you discover your inner diva. Will you be a Bollywood babe, Burlesque minx, Hip-Hop honey, Broadway star or Latino mama? Whichever you are, why not learn that specific workout first and you'll see that all you need to do is pack your doubts away, switch on your showbiz smile and come dancing...

Alison Pylkkänen
Editor of *Zest* magazine

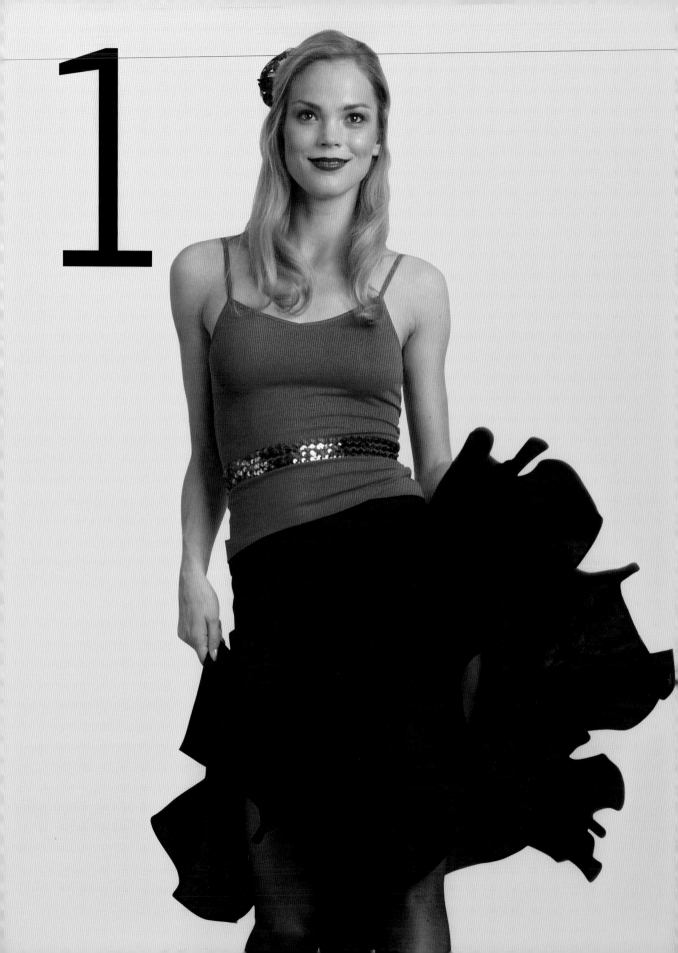

1

Getting Started

B y choosing this book, you're well on the way to discovering the body-boosting benefits of dance. But you might also be confused about where to begin. Should you start with a classic Broadway routine? Some Latin-inspired Salsa? Or a Bollywood, Burlesque or Hip Hop workout? Well, stress no more. On page 10, you'll find a six-question quiz designed to help you identify your perfect dance style. Answer the questions honestly, and the results will point you in the direction of a workout you'll love.

This chapter is also packed with information to help banish new-dancer nerves. If you think you're too inflexible or left-footed to dance, turn to page 9 and prepare to have your worries quashed. Dance is a fabulous way to tone the body, correct postural problems and boost confidence. You'll find more on the amazing benefits of dance on page 8.

Finally, this chapter will help you figure out what to wear when you work out. You don't need heaps of expensive equipment to dance, but a correctly-fitting pair of shoes and a few well-chosen props can make all the difference between an OK workout and a fabulous workout. So start reading and get ready to dance your way to fitness…

❛ Dance has amazing benefits – it tones your body, boosts confidence and helps to correct postural problems. ❜

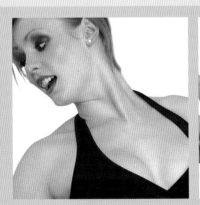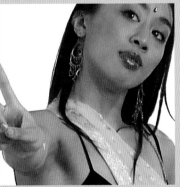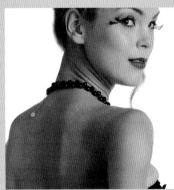

Why dance your way to fitness?

You can be forgiven for feeling nervous about dancing your way to fitness. Well, don't panic. To give you some inspiration before you start, here are five motivating reasons why dance is a great way to get fit.

1 It's great for the cardiovascular system

According to cardiac nurses, dance is an excellent exercise for keeping the heart healthy. Because it's aerobically challenging, a dance session will stimulate blood flow and pump freshly oxygenated blood through the arteries. This in turn helps to reduce the risk of high blood pressure, which lowers cholesterol levels and lessens the risk of heart disease. It will make you feel fabulous, too.

2 It calms overactive brains

If your life is ruled by an overactive brain, dance could be the perfect way to de-stress and help you relax. Researchers at the University College of Dance in Stockholm recently discovered that dance therapy is an effective way of calming down boys who suffer from ADHD (Attention Deficit Hyper Disorder), and of rehabilitating people who suffer from depression. If you're switched on 24/7 and often find yourself feeling stressed, try dancing – it will use up your excess energy, help you to relax and leave you happier and calmer than before.

3 It keeps you young

Dance could well be the perfect activity to keep you feeling young. In a recent study published in the *New England Journal of Medicine*, doctors discovered that dancing can help prevent the onset of dementia. Out of eleven physical activities, including swimming and cycling, dance was the only activity that benefited the brain. This was attributed to the cerebral rather than physical effects of dance. So if you want to keep your brain young and active, start learning some dance steps – the perfect way to give yourself a brain-boosting workout.

4 It's good for back problems

Many common postural problems, such as slouched shoulders and lower back pain, can be corrected by regularly stretching out the spine and developing core strength in the abdominals. The warm-up in this book, developed by physiotherapist and professional dancer Caroline Graham, will help to de-stress your back and train you to stand tall. Do it regularly enough and you'll be helping to keep your spine in tip-top shape.

5 It tones the body

Last but not least, dance is a brilliant all-over body toner. The routines in this book include walks, jumps, kicks, lunges, squats, thrusts and many other moves that you'd see in an aerobics, yoga or body conditioning class. Different movements work wonders on different parts of the body, but the great thing about dance is that the entire body gets a workout, without you even realizing it. Regular dancing will help you to increase your muscle tone and decrease your body fat. And you'll soon discover muscles you never knew you had!

Common worries quashed

Want to dance but worried you don't have the necessary grace, flexibility or coordination to pull it off? Everyone has doubts when they take up a new activity, but don't let a fear of failure put you off. Read on for some confidence-boosting tips.

1 'I'm too out of shape to dance'

You might not be as trim as a ballet dancer right now, but it's never too late to take up exercise and dance is a fabulous way to get fit and toned fast. Many of the routines in this book will take less than five minutes to do, so if you don't feel fit enough to repeat a routine just dance it once and then take a break by marching on the spot or stopping for a stretch. Varying the pace of your workout is an great way to build stamina. Before you know it, you'll be feeling stronger than ever.

2 'I've got two left feet'

Lots of people write themselves off as having two left feet. The truth is, if you can walk down the road using both legs, you'll be able to dance! Many of us have one side of the body that's more receptive to instruction than the other – this is a natural consequence of modern life and of being left- or right-handed. And while getting both sides of the body to work in sync might take a while, if you practise, you will get there in the end. To help you quash your worries, pick a song you absolutely love, turn it up loud and start moving. Before you know it, you'll be dancing.

3 'I'm not flexible enough'

Contrary to popular belief, you don't need to be super flexible to dance. If you warm up properly and stretch your muscles before you begin, you'll be able to perform the routines safely. If a routine features a kick and you can only lift your foot a few inches off the floor, this is absolutely fine – just give it a go rather than missing out the move all together. Dance is great for loosening muscles such as hamstrings and calves. The routines will elongate your arms and legs, meaning that over time, your flexibility is sure to increase and you'll look slimmer and leaner as a consequence.

4 'I don't have a dancer's physique'

What exactly is a dancer's physique? Curvy like J-Lo? Tiny like Kylie? Or muscle-bound like Madonna? These three women couldn't look more different if they tried. Yet all of them make dance a major focus of their shows and all of them look fabulous when they perform. When we dance, we use our arms, legs and faces to create a character and to draw people in – and any dancer will tell you that it's what you do with your body that counts, rather than what shape it is to begin with!

5 'I don't want to make a fool of myself'

Everyone worries about this from time to time, but sometimes we have to take a risk in order to get anywhere in life. If you don't have the confidence to dance in public yet, don't hit the club scene just now. Instead, clear a space in your bedroom, close the curtains and turn your favourite tune up loud. Spend a few weeks working through the routines in private. When you're ready to share your new skills, get your friends round and teach them how to do your favourite dance. Before you know it, you'll be rocking your local dancefloor with everyone following you.

What's your perfect dance style?

Answer a six-question quiz and find out

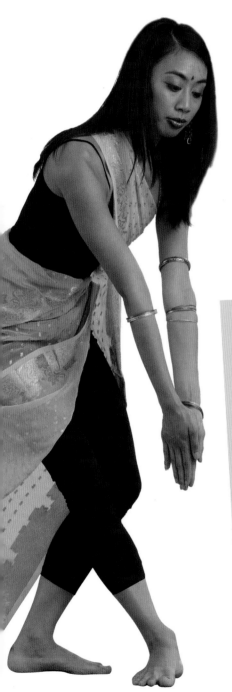

Before you throw yourself into your first workout, why not take five minutes to ID your perfect dance style? This book contains five different workouts and over time you should aim to try each workout at least once. To help you decide which routine to start with, take this six-question quiz. Simply work through the questions below, then total up your scores and check out the results panel on the next page. Your answers will point you in the direction of a specific dance routine. So before you lace up your dancing shoes and warm up, it's time to figure out what sort of dancer you really are, deep down!

1 Your friends are coming over for a girls' night in. To get ready for their arrival, do you:

A: Transform your lounge into a pampering palace and prepare your *Grease* DVD?

B: Glam yourself up, mix a jug of champagne cocktails and kick back with some sultry jazz music?

C: Slick back your hair, throw your jogging bottoms on and stick Christina Aguilera's latest album on your iPod?

D: Reinvent your living room by draping bright and beautiful fabrics over the sofas, and ordering in some Asian cuisine?

E: Mix some salsa and guacamole, open a pack of tortillas and put your tequila in the freezer?

2 You've saved £1,000 for a dream holiday. Where do you go?

A: New York – nothing beats the energy of a weekend in the Big Apple.

B: Paris – a city for lovers and culture junkies. It's your home from home.

C: Los Angeles – it's got malls and A-listers galore. What more could a girl need?

D: Delhi – the crowds, the colours, the craziness – it's right up your street.

E: Buenos Aires – a buzzing, exciting South American city.

3 The last great workout you did consisted of:

A: An old-school aerobics class, complete with grapevines, mini routines and leg warmers.

B: A 60-minute session in the swimming pool and spa. Effective but elegant too.

C: An old-fashioned jog through the park, fuelled by pumping tunes on your MP3 player.

D: A super-fun belly-dancing class. You're always surprised by how much it makes you sweat.

E: An hour of yoga, Pilates or Body Balance. Perfect for stretching and toning your limbs.

4 Your friend wants to take you the theatre for your birthday. If all these shows were on, which one would you choose?

A: *The Producers* – the showgirls; the costumes; the bad jokes! Perfect.

B: *Chicago* – the fishnets; the smoky eyes. An irresistible combination.

C: *Footloose* – the funky routines; the jumps through mid-air. You love it.

D: *Bombay Dreams* – the glitz; the glamour; the bootyliciousness of it all!

E: *Dirty Dancing* – you've waited years to see 'that lift' live on stage.

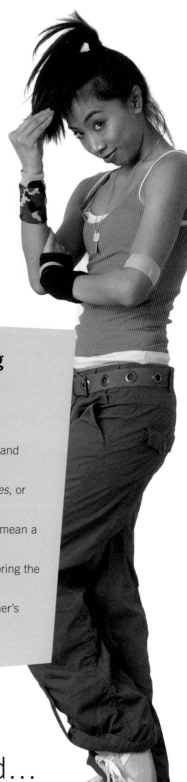

5 You're going out partying with your friends. What do you wear?

A: Black trousers and a 'look at me' top, with dancefloor-friendly pumps.

B: A little black dress with fishnets and killer heels. It works every time.

C: Combats and a funky top with a statement bandana in your hair.

D: A bright pink dress with sexy beads and extra-sparkly accessories.

E: A full-skirted dress with a flower in your hair. You like to feel pretty.

6 It's your anniversary and your man is planning an extra-special date. Where are you secretly hoping to end up?

A: On the dancefloor at your local 70s club. You're buzzing with excitement and want to dance the night away.

B: At the cinema, watching Marilyn do her thing in *Gentlemen Prefer Blondes*, or another fabulous old movie.

C: At an all-night party with the rest of your crew. Romance doesn't have to mean a quiet night in.

D: At the movies watching the latest tear-jerking romantic comedy. He can bring the tissues!

E: At a busy, old-school dancehall in the city centre. You'll join in the beginner's lesson and then watch the other couples dance.

Now add up your totals.
If you scored...

Mostly As: Broadway babe

You're a high-energy lady who loves being dazzled by bright lights and fancy footwork. Films such as *Fame*, *Saturday Night Fever* and *Footloose* are your favourites, and you're always the first one to dance when the DJ cues up an old-school floor-filler. You love going to see shows and you'd kill to know how to do a pirouette. Turn to page 58 and get started on our exclusive Broadway workout – you'll soon have your friends begging for an encore!

You should also try: Hip Hop and Burlesque – you've got the energy needed for Hip Hop, and the confidence required for Burlesque.

Mostly Bs: Burlesque temptress

You're elegant, sexy and know how to entertain and socialize in style. You enjoy being the centre of attention and feel super-confident when dressed in your trusty LBD and sky-high stilettos. You love dancing because it gives you an opportunity to flaunt your confident side and show off your sexy curves. Forget sweat – you want to be drenched in smoky eyeshadow, barely-there satin and seductive diamonds when you work out. Turn to page 120 and indulge in our Burlesque routine. If it's good enough for The Pussycat Dolls…

You should also try: Latin and Broadway – you've got the grace and style for Broadway routines, and the go-getting mentality for Latin dance.

Mostly Cs: Hip Hop diva

You're a funky, pumped-up girl who loves working hard, playing hard and having fun. You come alive when the music is loud, and whether you're partying to new tunes, old-school R 'n' B or vintage Madonna, you love nothing more than shaking your funky stuff on the dancefloor. You're a straight-talking, no-frills girl and you'd rather get out there and enjoy life than spend hours getting ready for it. Turn to page 36 and get cracking on our Hip Hop routine. Beyoncé had better watch out.

You should also try: Bollywood and Broadway – you've got the energy for our pumping Bollywood workout, and you've got the show-stopping stance needed for Broadway.

Mostly Ds: Bollywood star

You're a sophisticated woman who appreciates the bright, beautiful and bold things in life. You're a romantic at heart and you love seeing new places, meeting new people and experiencing new cultures. You're not afraid to question life and probe beyond the surface to find out why things happen they way they do. When it comes to working out, you like to use your body in a womanly, holistic way – no treadmills and cross-trainers for a free spirit like you! Turn to page 98 and try our Bollywood workout. You'll soon be shimmying and jumping your way to fitness!

You should also try: Burlesque and Latin – indulge your sexy side with a Burlesque dance, and harness your creative energy in a Latin routine.

Mostly Es: Latino lady

You're a liberated, free spirit who loves flirting, talking and partying with all the interesting people you meet. You'd rather eat lightly and sip cocktails than sit down to a plate of comfort food. When it comes to working out, you prefer laid-back exercises that let you breathe fresh air, socialize and have fun – no sweaty gym classes and heavy weights for you! Tango and Salsa dance appeals to your inquisitive nature, so turn to page 80 to get started on our Latin workout. J-Lo will be quaking in her high heels.

You should also try: Broadway and Burlesque – you'll love the ladylike chic of our Broadway routine, and thrive on the flirty, fun moves in the Burlesque workout.

First steps: essential dance kit

Kylie does it in hotpants, Madonna does it in cowboy boots and Beyoncé does it in super-short dresses. But whichever way you look at it, dance's flexible dress code is a brilliant thing. Unlike tennis, golf and many other sports that women love, you don't need to invest hundreds of pounds on kit or equipment before you hit the dancefloor. You can literally throw on a pair of sweat pants and a vest and get going. This makes dance accessible to everyone and means you can spend just a few minutes getting ready for your workout.

However, it is worth investing in an outfit that will make you feel fabulous while you dance. Dancing in front of a mirror can boost your performance 100 per cent and if you like what you see staring back at you, you'll stand taller, execute your movements with more passion, smile and have more fun. It's also important to wear the correct footwear for the dance style. So before you throw yourself into a workout, check out the following breakdown of essential kit for each dance style in this book.

Broadway

Must have:
A good pair of jazz trainers
No show dancer's kit bag is complete without a pair of lace-up dance trainers. Specialist dancewear company Bloch makes a fantastic shoe called the Slingshot <www.blochworld.com> and Nike has recently launched its super-lightweight Zoom Danzante trainer <www.nikewomen.com>. Both styles support the ankle but have flexible soles specifically designed to allow your foot to flex while dancing.

Could have:
Hats, canes and heels
There are no hard and fast rules when it comes to Broadway costumes. The kids in *Fame* wear leg warmers and leotards; the murderesses in *Chicago* flaunt fishnets, top hats and canes. Invest in a few choice props that work for you. Once you're confident with the routine, swap your trainers for low, square-heeled shoes to give yourself a height boost. Don't forget the number one accessory in dance: you. Point your fingers and toes, stand tall, and let your body do the talking.

Burlesque

Must have:
A pair of heeled shoes
Aside from being natural leg-lengtheners, heels tilt the pelvis and make it easier to perform Burlesque routines. Stilettos are a staple of every showgirl's costume cupboard, but until you're confident, dance in a trusty old pair of heels that don't hurt your feet.

Could have:
Long gloves, a corset and red lipstick
Some Burlesque performers dress in a cutesy, girly way; others vamp it up with painted lips and sexy props. At first, you'll be more interested in learning the steps than styling yourself, but to increase the fun factor, invest in some long gloves or a waist-tightening corset. Fans, false eyelashes and a glamorous top will work wonders for your confidence too, so don't be afraid to dress up. Costume is a great way to speed up your transformation from novice to performer, so grab something sparkly and set your Burlesque spirit free.

Bollywood

Must have:
Bare feet
The Bollywood routine in this book draws on traditional, ancient forms of dance that Indian women used to perform when harvesting crops in the field. In keeping with its natural origins, it's best to dance Bhangra moves barefoot. However, if you've only got access to carpeted surfaces, wear trainers instead. Carpet burns certainly won't help you feel liberated!

Could have:
A brightly coloured dress and headscarf
Bollywood dance is a celebration of life. So why not throw a colourful top or floaty dress over black leggings and a vest top, to bring some sunshine to the routine? If you're feeling creative, consider buying fabric to make your very own dress (or at least a head-scarf), and put this on for the dance. Many local markets have fabric stalls that sell chiffon, silk and other funky fabrics at low cost.

Latin

Must have:
A sexy pair of heels
To maximize your chances of capturing that South American spirit, consider buying a proper pair of dance heels and wearing them once you've familiarized yourself with the routine in this book. The elegant Tara Latin Shoe at Freeds of London <www.freed oflondon. com/cat/index.php> is a sexy silver shoe that would work a treat. High-street stores will also be brimming with alternatives.

Could have:
Fake tan, pony tail and full skirt
Sexy hair works wonders in Latin dance. Whatever the length of your hair, wear it down and let it bounce around naturally as you move. Loose hair, plus a smidgen of fake tan on your skin, will give you an extra confidence boost and help to unleash your Latin spirit as you dance. A full skirt will look fabulous when you move.

Hip Hop

Must have:
Trainers with proper support
When it comes to Hip Hop dance, anything goes. But don't let ultra- laid-back Hip Hop stars lead you in a dangerous direction: baggy clothing is fine, but your shoes should be laced up tightly and offer good ankle support, so that no extra pressure is exerted on your foot and ankle joints while you dance. The Nike Zoom Danzante trainer is a great shoe for Hip Hop dance. Other leading brands, such as Reebok <www.reebokstore. co.uk>, Puma <www.puma.com> and Adidas <www.adidas.com> also offer a range of shoes suitable for dancing.

Could have:
Combats, sweat bands and visor
There's no such thing as too much bling for Hip Hop stars. If you want to be like Missy Elliot, head to the high street and stock up on chains, visors, sweat bands and whatever funky accessories take your fancy. It will help you unleash your inner diva and make you feel ghetto-fabulous!

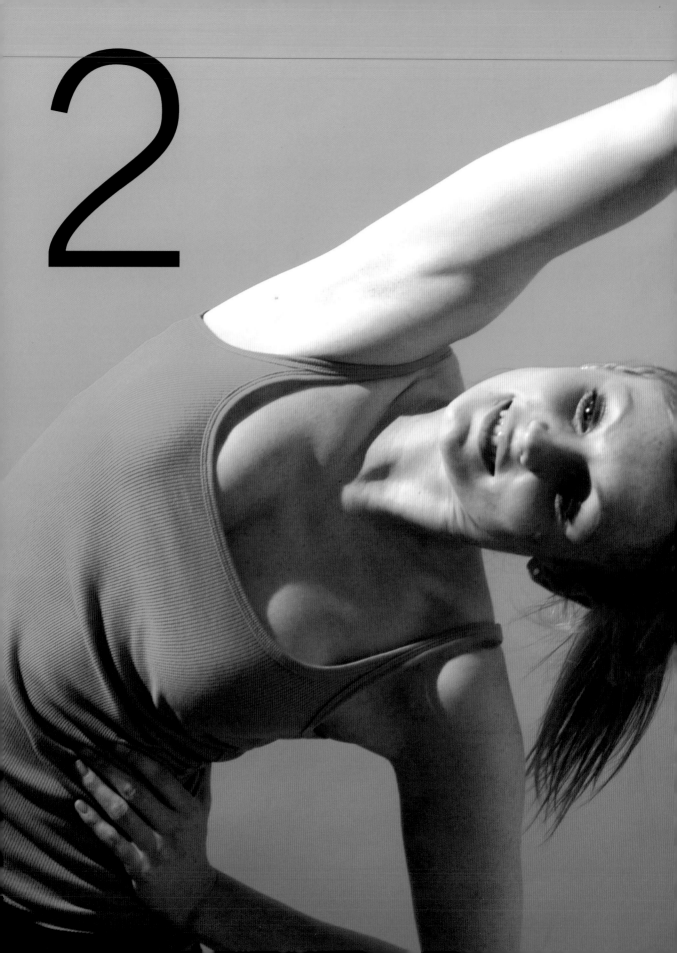

2

The Warm Up

You've charged your iPod, filled your water bottle and sent your flatmates to the shops. Congratulations – you're almost ready to dance! But before you begin, it's important to spend some time systematically warming up all of your muscles. Professional dancers will always follow a warm-up of some kind and if you skip this vital stage, you run the risk of developing an injury. To help you avoid this, on the following pages the easy-to-follow warm-up plan will gently raise your pulse rate, get your circulation going and prepare your body for the physical challenge that's about to follow.

The great thing about dance warm-ups is that they are actually a lot of fun. Some teachers spend as long as 40 minutes warming up their students before they teach a routine – and this is in a class that's just 60 minutes long! A warm up of this length might sound like ages, but extended warm-ups give students the perfect opportunity to forget their worries, slip into 'performance mode' and work out exactly how flexible, strong and coordinated their bodies are feeling. Every day is different, and it's important not to push yourself if your body is resisting. Dance is an artistic form and there's nothing artistic about collapsing on the floor because you simply didn't listen when your limbs said no. In fact, even if you are super-fit, you must make sure that you are working within your body's natural limitations, and not pushing yourself too hard. To make sure you exercise safely and get your workout off to a great start, see the section on Preventing Injury on page 18 before you move a muscle.

> **A proper warm up will enable you to forget your worries, slip into "performance mode" and work out how flexible, strong and coordinated your body is feeling.**

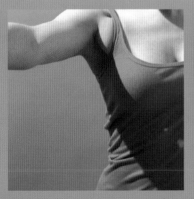
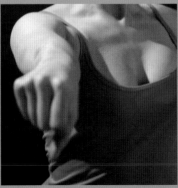
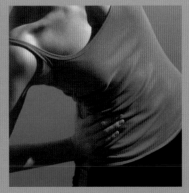

Preventing injury

Consider these five points before you hit the warm-up mat

1

Existing injuries
Don't ignore swollen ankles or sore knees. Dance is a high-impact activity and it can put pressure on your joints. Make sure that your joints are correctly aligned. Any movement that feels really unnatural – or that puts you into a difficult position – is probably going to misalign your joints. Don't force yourself. Seek advice from your doctor if you have any worries.

2

Pain
If you suddenly experience pain whilst warming up or dancing, stop. The routines in this book will challenge you and some movements will feel odd at first. But if you experience any shooting pains, ease off and start cooling down straight away. Do as much as your body allows you to, but don't fight through pain.

3

Your physical capabilities
Everyone using this book will have different physical strengths and weaknesses. You may even have old injuries that occasionally give you trouble. Over time, regular exercise can strengthen your weak spots, but initially there's no point pushing it. Honour your body's needs. This means working within your own physical capabilities – no one else's.

4

Post-workout assessment
Do you feel pleasantly stiff or painfully achy the day after a workout? A slight ache in the body can be satisfying – it feels like proof that you've worked hard. But discomfort isn't good. If you're too tired to walk up the stairs the day after dancing, you've been working too hard and you should ease off next time.

5

Overall workout experience
If you're smiling and laughing the whole way through your workout, you're probably doing things right. But if you're grimacing through gritted teeth, something is wrong. Be aware, though, that adrenaline released during exercise can mask natural pain receptors. To counteract this problem, stop for a water break every ten minutes and gently give your body an all-over stretch.

How to use this book

● All of the moves and dance sequences in the following chapters are suitable for beginners. So even if you've never danced in your life, you will be able to get these moves right after a bit of practice.

● Every move is explained using a combination of pictures and captions. The text offers detailed instruction on what to do with your body and the pictures will help guide you to the right position.

● Dotted throughout the text are a series of 'pro tips'. These tips come direct from leading choreographers, and they are designed to give you an expert push in the right direction. Each workout has a 'killer move' – a move that sums up the essense of the dance style, and which is perfect for dazzling your friends with!

● The great thing is that this book is yours to keep forever – so you don't have to worry about getting your legs and arms right on your first attempt. Keep practising and you will succeed.

Dancing at the right pace for your fitness level and choosing the right music

Once you've got the hang of the moves, you'll be ready to string them all together and dance. To help you dance at a pace appropriate for your fitness level, every routine in this book – including the warm-up – can be executed at one of three different levels.

Level 1: Getting fit – if you're new to exercise, start here.

Don't be afraid! The routines in this book are beginner-friendly and perfect for those who are gym-phobic. You should dance to a track from the Getting Fit playlist at the end of each chapter. As your stamina builds, you'll want to push yourself more, so then you can move on to…

Level 2: Fighting fit – if you're of average fitness, start here.

You probably already exercise twice a week and you can hold your own in a fitness studio. So, choose a track from Fighting Fit playlist and when this stops being challenging, bump yourself up to…

Level 3: Super-fit – if you're extra strong and fit, start here.

You probably work out three to four times per week and have strong core and leg muscles. You need to dance to up-tempo Super-fit tracks and do the highest number of repetitions and sets in the warm-up section of this book.

The important thing to remember is that the moves are the same whether you're doing Level 1, Level 2 or Level 3. The only thing that's different is the number of repetitions, the aerobic intensity of the workouts and the tempo of the music. If you're not sure what your fitness level is, follow the warm-up workout at the Fighting Fit level – then stay there or take the level down or up depending on how easy or tough you find the challenge.

The warm-up workout

The workout programme on pages 20–35 works every major muscle group in the body and will prepare you for whichever dance routine you choose to follow first. Incorporating cardiovascular work, ballet stretches and core strength exercises, the warm-up should take you 20–30 minutes to get through. The exact length of time will depend on your fitness level and the number of repetitions you complete. It will also depend on the pace of the music you choose. But don't rush. Dancing is your time to work on your body and mind, so think of it as valuable 'me time'. Pace yourself, drink plenty of water and enjoy the experience.

Kit tip: *If you've got a yoga or dance mat, you might like to use it for the core strength exercises. And if you're using a carpeted surface, wear trainers throughout the warm-up to protect yourself from carpet burns. However, if you're dancing on a wooden floor or lino, feel free to warm up barefoot. This will help with your balance and come in handy when you reach the ballet section of the routine.*

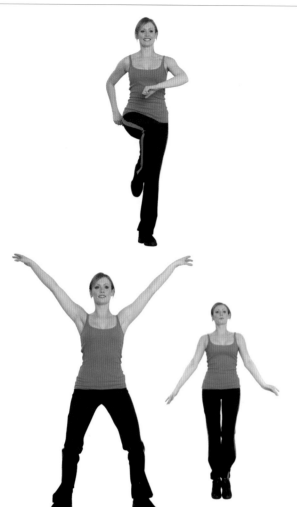

1 Marching on the spot

March on the spot for 8 counts. Keep your fists clenched and hold your arms up to chest level. Keep your back nice and straight.

Getting fit: Keep your feet low and march at a steady pace. Complete 2 sets of 8 repetitions.

Fighting fit: Make your step more of a jog than a march, by lifting your feet higher off the floor. Complete 4 sets of 8 repetitions.

Super-fit: Start off jogging on the spot, but by the second set, lift your legs higher, so your thigh is parallel to the floor and your calves are pointing down. Complete 6 sets of 8 repetitions.

2 Star jumps

1. Stand with both feet together, hands by your side. Jump your feet apart as far as they can go, keeping your knees slightly bent. At the same time, extend your arms sideways until parallel to the floor.
2. Then jump your feet back together and bring your arms back by your sides.

Getting fit: 8 star jumps.

Fighting fit: 16 star jumps.

Super-fit: 24 star jumps.

3 Forward lunges

1. Stand with both feet together.
2. Lunge your left foot forwards and jump your right foot back. At the same time, clench your fists and plunge your right arm forwards and bring your left arm back.
3. Then do it again, this time with your right foot and left arm coming forwards, and your right arm and left foot moving back.

Getting fit: 8 reps.

Fighting fit: 16 reps.

Super-fit: 24 reps.

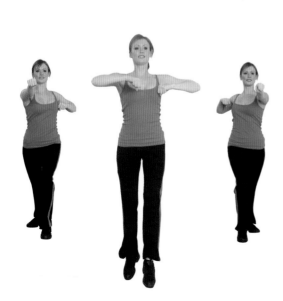

> **PRO TIP:** This move requires opposite actions for arms and legs, so try it in slow motion until you get the hang of it. It's worth persevering, because the punches are great for toning your upper arms and the jumps are great for toning your legs. Your heart rate will get a good boost too!

4 Sideways jumps and punches

1. Stand on the spot with your feet together.
2. Make 4 consecutive jumps towards the left side of the room. As you move, punch your left arm out in the direction you are moving.
3. Then reverse the movement and jump 4 times towards the right side of the room. As you move, punch your right arm out in the direction you are moving.

Getting fit: 2 sets of 4 jumps in each direction.
Fighting fit: 4 sets of 4 jumps in each direction.
Super-fit: 6 sets of 4 jumps in each direction.

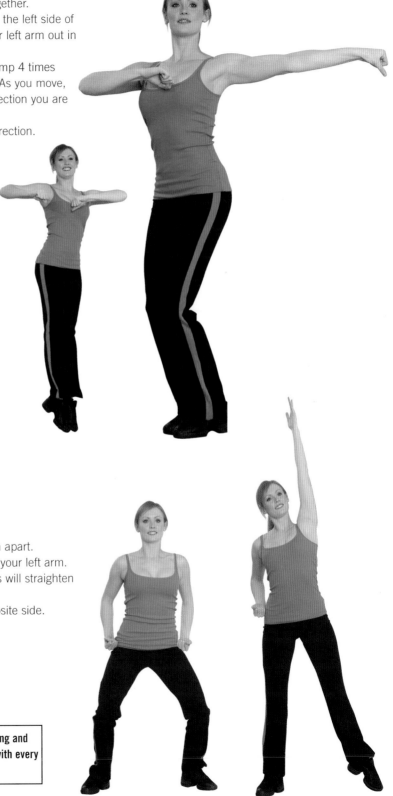

5 Side step and reach

1. Stand with your feet shoulder-width apart.
2. Bend your knees slightly and raise your left arm. Stretch over to your right. Both legs will straighten as you move.
3. Repeat this movement on the opposite side.

Getting fit: 4 reps in each direction (alternating left and right).
Fighting fit: 8 reps in each direction (alternating left and right).
Super-fit: 12 reps in each direction (alternating left and right).

> **PRO TIP:** This move is excellent for trimming and toning your waist, so stretch a bit further with every repetition to maximize the benefits.

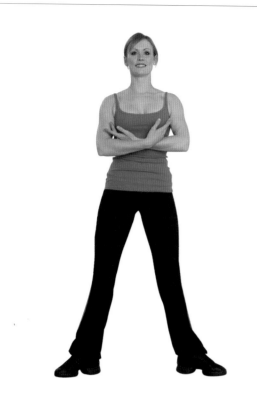

Stretching exercises

6 Plié with stretch

1. Stand with your feet shoulder-width apart. Turn your toes out. Cross your arms in front of your body.
2. Bend your knees and sink down as if you were sitting on an imaginary chair. Keep your back straight. As you bend your knees, open your arms and stretch them out to the side.
3. Then stretch your legs and stand up. As you do this inhale. Stretch your arms up to the ceiling and point your fingers.
4. Exhale and bend your knees again to repeat the move.

Getting fit: 2 reps.
Fighting fit: 4 reps.
Super-fit: 6 reps.

> **PRO TIP:** Don't force your body down too low. This is a gentle stretch, designed to wake up your spine and legs. So if you can't get your thighs parallel to the floor, don't worry. Your flexibility and strength will increase with time and practice.

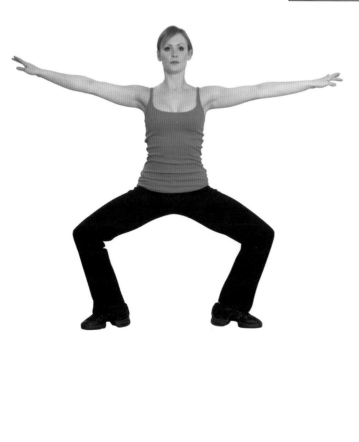

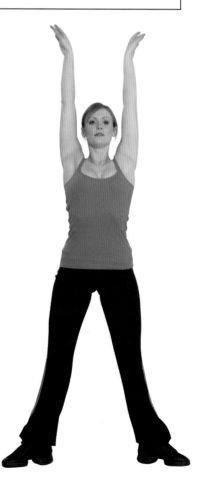

7 Shoulder circles and knee bends

1. Stand with your legs 1m apart and your shoulders relaxed.
2. Bend your knees and hold for 1 second.
3. As you straighten your legs, roll your shoulders up and backwards. Stretch your arms out slightly and keep tension in your hands.
3. Straighten your legs and hold for 1 second.
4. Once you get the hang of this movement, keep alternating between bent knees and straight legs.
5. Now reverse your arm movement so your shoulders are rolling forwards.

Getting fit: 2 backwards / 2 forwards.
Fighting fit: 4 backwards / 4 forwards.
Super-fit: 6 backwards / 6 forwards.

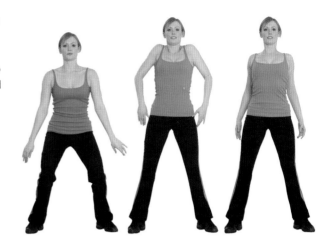

8 Head and neck stretches

Front and back
1. Face the front of the room. Keeping your body still, tilt your head forwards so you are looking at the floor.
2. Bring your head back to centre.
3. Tilt your head back so you are looking at the ceiling.

Side to side
1. Face the front of the room. Keeping your body still and eyes to the front, tilt your head to the right-hand side, on a diagonal angle.
2. Bring your head back to centre.
3. Now tilt it to the left-hand side, on a diagonal angle.

All fitness levels: 2 rolls to the front and back; 2 rolls to the left and right.

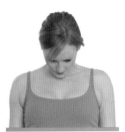

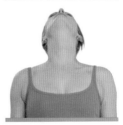

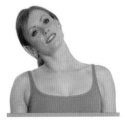

PRO TIP: When you tilt your head back, don't force it back too far as this can constrict blood flow. Just tilt it back far enough to look up at the ceiling. If anything feels uncomfortable, ease off.

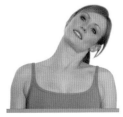

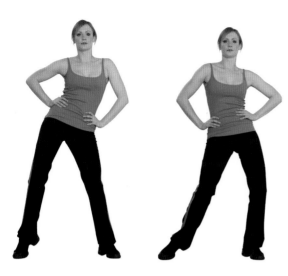

9 Hip rolls

1. Stand with your feet hip-width apart and place your hands on your hips.
2. Roll your hips in a clockwise direction, as if you were drawing a circle with your bottom.
3. As you roll your hips, your knees will naturally bend and straighten. This is fine – let your hips lead and your legs will follow.
4. Repeat the move in an anticlockwise direction.

All fitness levels: 4 rolls clockwise; 4 rolls anticlockwise.

> **PRO TIP:** Hip rolls are brilliant for loosening up your lower-body. The first hip roll of the day should be small, but as you work through the reps, increase the intensity of the movement, so that by your eighth hip roll, you are drawing a big circle with your hips. This will come in handy when you start working on the Burlesque and Latin routines later on.

10 Side body bend

1. Stand with your feet shoulder-width apart.
2. Keeping your right hand on your right hip, bring your left arm over your head and stretch to the right as far as you can go.
3. Hold the position for 10 seconds and release. Then reverse the movement torepeat on the left-hand side.

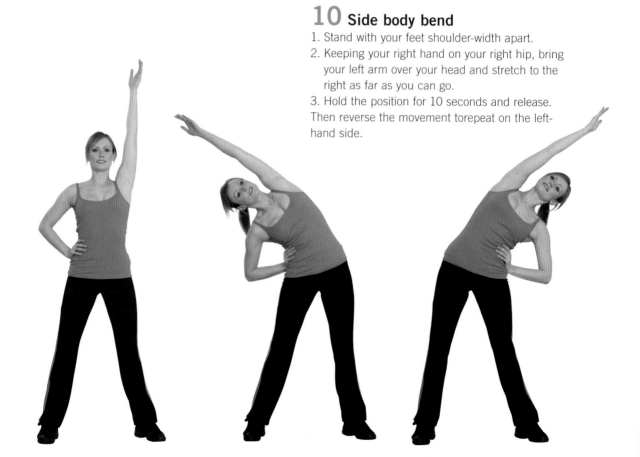

11 Forward stretch

1. Stand with your legs as far apart as is comfortable (this could be shoulder-width apart or it could be 1m apart). Raise your arms above your head. Bend forwards from your hips and let your body hang down towards the floor.
2. Hold the position for 10 seconds and release.

> **PRO TIP:** You don't have to keep your legs straight and get your fingers all the way to the floor for the forward stretch to have an impact. Bend your knees if keeping them straight is painful, and rest your hands on your ankles or calves if this is easier. The stretch is excellent for your quads and glutes, and it gives you a nice chance to relax and take some deep breaths before moving on.

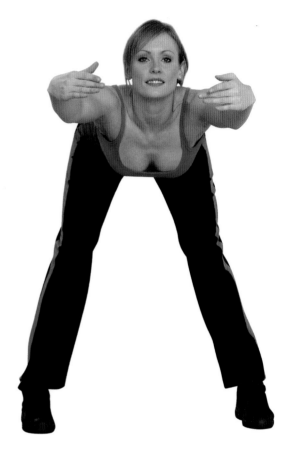

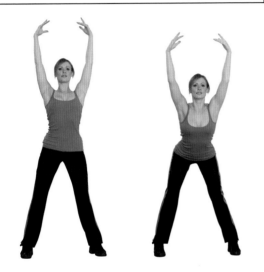

12 Standing calf stretch

For this stretch you might like to lean against a wall or door to help you maintain your balance.

1. Step your left foot forwards and keep your right foot directly behind.
2. Bend your left knee and lean forwards. Keep your right heel on the floor and hold the pose for 20 seconds.
3. Reverse the movement to repeat on the right calf.

> **PRO TIP:** When you hold the pose it might seem like a long time, but it takes this long for your muscle to really relax. Breathe deeply as you hold the pose, and focus on the fabulously toned legs you are going to have after a few weeks of working through this routine!

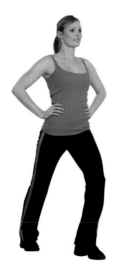

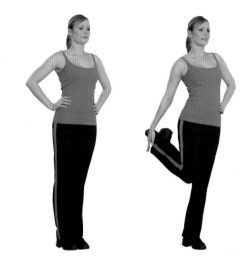

13 Standing quad stretch

1. Stand with both feet together with your hands resting on your hips.
2. Stretch your right arm down. Reach behind you and pick up your right foot.
3. Bring your foot as near to your buttock as you can get it. You will feel a stretch in your front of your thigh. Allow your hips to tilt forwards. Hold the position for 20 seconds.
4. Reverse the movement to repeat on your left leg.

> **PRO TIP:** Don't worry if you feel your lower back arching slightly as you carry out this move – that's normal. And if you can only lift your leg halfway up to your buttock, that's fine too. You'll still be stretching and toning your thighs, which is the point of this move.

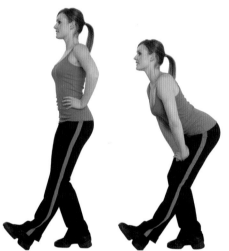

14 Standing hamstring stretch

1. Step your left foot in front of your right foot. Dig your right heel into the floor and point your toes to the ceiling.
2. Keeping your back flat, lean forwards from your hips and stick your bottom out. Bend your right leg if you need to.
3. Press down on the top of your left thigh and lean forwards with your torso. Hold the pose for 20 seconds.
4. Reverse this movement to repeat on your right leg.

15 Back stretch

1. Lie down on your stomach.
2. Place your hands on the floor next to your shoulders, palms facing down.
3. Lift your upper body off the floor until your arms are straight. Hold the position for 10 seconds.

Getting fit: 1 rep.
Fighting fit: 2 reps.
Super-fit: 3 reps.

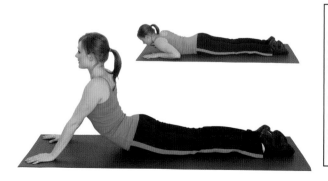

> **PRO TIP:** If you've got a strong and flexible back, straighten your arms all the way and really go for this stretch. But if you can't get your torso very high off the floor and you have to keep your arms bent, don't worry. Your spine will get stronger and more flexible as you progress, so take it easy to start with. And as your fitness level increases, you'll be able to hold the position for longer. Remember to breathe as you execute this move. Inhale deeply on your way up, and slowly exhale on your way down.

16 Cat back stretch

1. From the position in exercise 15, move on to all fours. Your shins and hands should be on the floor.
2. Suck your tummy in and arch your back towards the ceiling. Hold for 3 seconds.
3. Then stick your bottom out, lower your back and arch your upper spine. Hold for 3 seconds.

All fitness levels: Repeat this move 4 times.

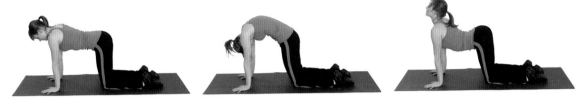

17 Sweeping stretch

1. Sit on the floor with your legs stretched out in front of you.
2. Raise your arms straight above your head.
3. Relax your arms down by your sides and then gently sweep them forwards along the side of your legs. When you reach your toes, scoop your arms up and start again.

All fitness levels: 3 reps.

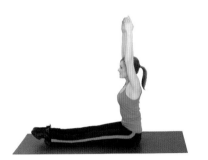

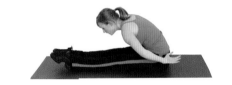

> **PRO TIP:** Stretches (exercises 17, 18 and 19) are great for opening up your hip joints. Don't push yourself too much – if you've never done yoga or dance before, you might not be able to get your legs very low on the floor. But give it a go. The more you practise, the easier the moves will become.

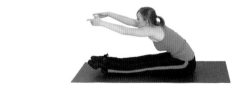

18 Hip opener

1. Sit on your floor with your legs bent and the soles of your feet pressed together in front of you.
2. Place your hands on your feet.
3. Gently push down on your ankles.

All fitness levels: 3 reps.

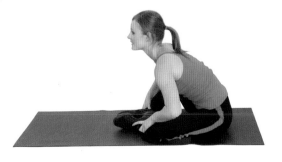

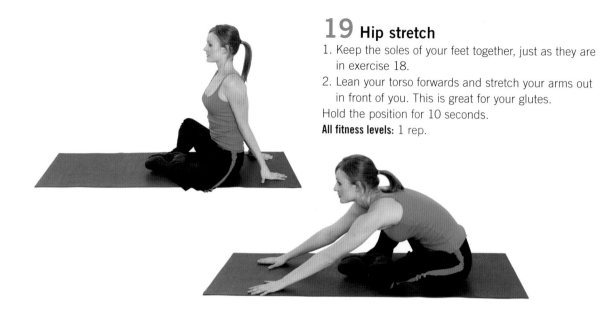

19 Hip stretch

1. Keep the soles of your feet together, just as they are in exercise 18.
2. Lean your torso forwards and stretch your arms out in front of you. This is great for your glutes.

Hold the position for 10 seconds.

All fitness levels: 1 rep.

Ballet-style exercises

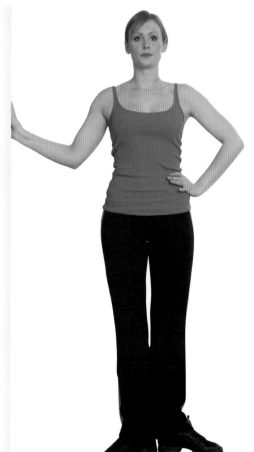

20 Toe stretch in first position

1. Stand sideways-on to a wall and place your right hand against it. Put your left hand on your hip.
2. Place your toes in 'first position', which means the heels are together; toes are pointing outwards.
3. Point your left foot in front of you, then to the side, then behind you.
4. Repeat the sequence with the right leg, with the left hand against the wall.

> **PRO TIP:** The moves in exercises 20 and 21 are excellent for restoring balance to your body, increasing coordination and getting you used to pointing your toes. If you've got a window sill or table edge that could double as a barre, use it. If not, hold on to the wall for support.

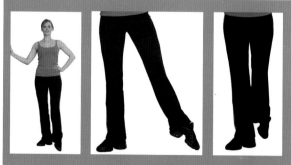

21 Plié in first position

1. Keeping your feet in first position, bend your knees as much as you can without taking your heels off the floor.
2. As you bend your knees, let your left arm rise up to hip level.
3. As you rise up and straighten your legs, bring your left arm back to your side.
4. Repeat the move, except this time let your heels come off the floor. This will allow your knees to bend more, and give you more of a stretch in the thighs. It's known as a full plié. Repeat each plié twice.
5. Repeat the sequence with your left arm against the wall, raising the right arm.

Repeat the pliés as above, but with feet in second position and third position.

Second position: Feet are shoulder-width apart and your toes are facing outwards.

Third position: Stand with one foot slightly in front of the other, so your feet are making a V-shape.

> **PRO TIP:** If your knees make a popping sound as you go down into a full plié, don't panic. It's not a bad sound – it's simply caused by oxygen moving around your kneecap and it's nothing to worry about. However if you experience pain at any point, ease off straight away.

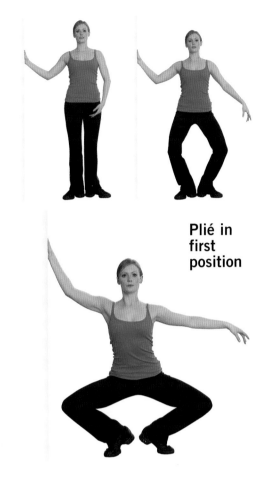

Plié in first position

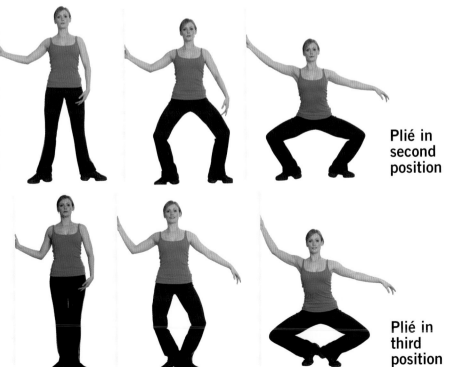

Plié in second position

Plié in third position

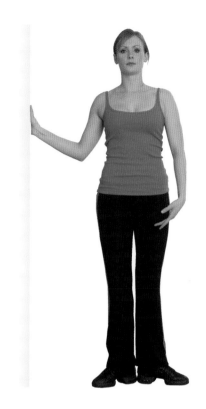
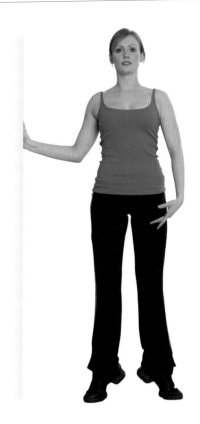

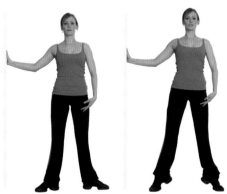

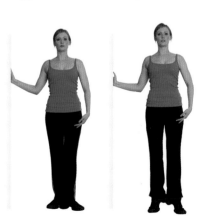

22 Rises

In first position:

1. Keep your feet together with your toes facing outwards.
2. Rise up on the balls of your feet and hold the position for 5 seconds.

In second position:

1. Stand with your feet shoulder-width apart, toes facing outwards.
2. Rise up on the balls of your feet and hold the position for 5 seconds.

In third position:

1. Stand with your left foot slightly in front of your right right foot, so your toes are pointing outwards in a V-shape.
2. Rise up on the balls of your feet and hold the position for 5 seconds.

PRO TIP: Rises are really good for strengthening your ankles. They also help with balance. Rest one arm against the wall, or hold a barre to help with balance, but over time, aim to let go of the surface and let your arms support you instead. Each of these rises should be done 4 times for all fitness levels.

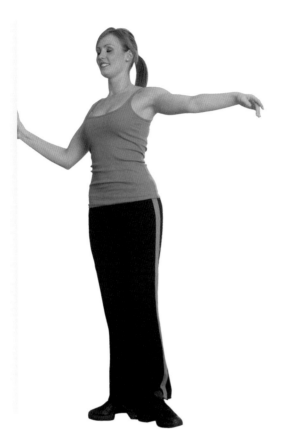

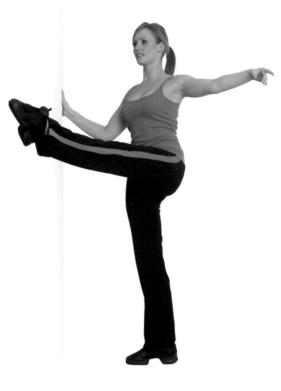

23 Front and back kicks

1. Rest your right hand against a wall or hold on to a barre.
2. Stretch your left arm out to the side.
3. Gently swing your left foot forwards and backwards in one continuous motion.
4. Repeat this move 4 times backwards and forwards. Turn around and repeat in the opposite direction – so your left arm will be against the wall and your right leg will be moving.

PRO TIP: Point your toes as you move your leg and keep your core muscles tight – this will help you stay balanced. Don't aim to kick your leg really high on your first attempt. It is better to start with low kicks and build up to a high level, than to injure yourself on your first attempt.

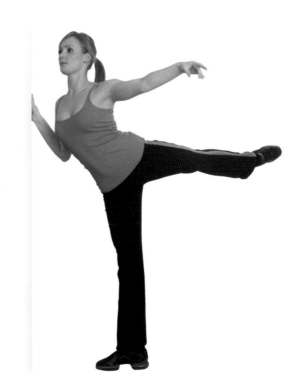

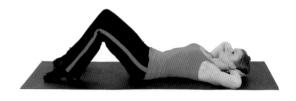

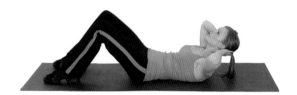

Core strength exercises

24 Crunch

1. Lie on the floor with your knees bent, feet flat on the floor.
2. Place your hands behind your head, elbows bent.
3. Pull in your abdominal muscles and push your lower back on to the floor.
4. Gently curl up so your shoulders come off the floor, then relax back down.

Getting fit: 10 reps.
Fighting fit: 15 reps.
Super-fit: 20 reps.

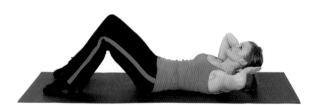

25 Half crunch

This move is exactly the same as before, except this time you lift your body slightly higher off the floor and split the movement into 2 phases.

1. Lie on the floor with your knees bent, feet flat on the floor.
2. Place your hands behind your head, elbows bent.
3. Pull in your abdominal muscles and push your lower back on to the floor.
4. Lift your head off the floor and hold for 1 count.
5. Lift your shoulders off the floor and hold for 1 count.

Getting fit: 4 reps.
Fighting fit: 7 reps.
Super-fit: 10 reps.

If you've got energy left at the end of the half crunches and want to give your tummy some extra toning, add another set of the normal crunches to your routine.

Getting fit: 10 reps.
Fighting fit: 15 reps.
Super-fit: 20 reps.

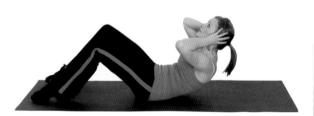

> **PRO TIP:** When doing sit-ups, it's tempting to lift your upper body all the way off the floor, so your torso is at a right angle to your legs. But there's no need to do this. Full body sit-ups might feel good, but they won't deliver the goods when it comes to toning your core area. So don't waste energy and breath sitting all the way up. Instead, keep the lower back in contact with the floor at all times and make your movements slow and controlled instead.

Press-ups

26 Wall press-up

1. Stand with your feet away from the wall, toes facing the wall. The wall should be slightly too far for the hands to reach.
2. Bend your elbows and lean forwards. Then push yourself back as you straighten your arms.

PRO TIP: Press-ups can be difficult, so to get started, work with the wall for 10 reps. The further away you stand, the more of a challenge the move will be – stand 1m away to give yourself a tough challenge, or 0.5m away to make the move slightly easier. If you're nervous about trying a full press-up on the floor, this approach is great for building your confidence gradually. And once you're doing a half or full press-up, don't force yourself to get your nose all the way to the floor. Even moving just a little way will get your triceps and pecs working, and will reap big benefits.

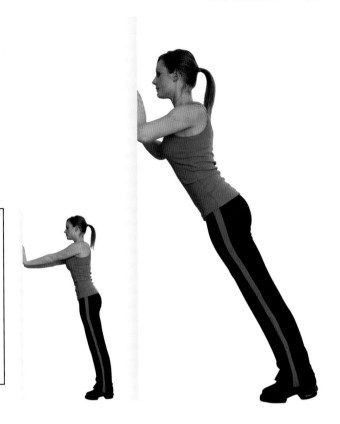

27 Half press-up

1. On your hands and knees, place your hands on the ground, a little wider than shoulder-width apart. Cross your ankles behind you.
2. Pull in your stomach muscles and bend the elbows, allowing the body to drop down towards the floor.
3. Push back up and straighten your arms.

Getting fit: 1 set of 5 wall press-ups and 5 half press-ups.
Fighting fit: 2 sets of 8 wall press-ups and 8 half press-ups.
Super-fit: 3 sets of 10 wall press-ups and 10 half press-ups.

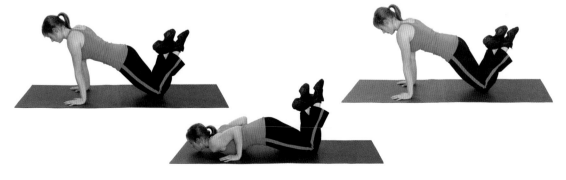

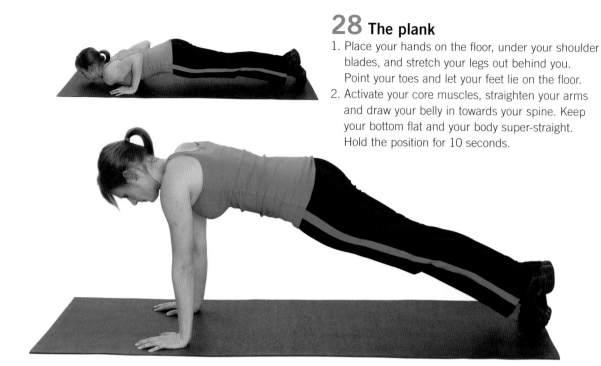

28 The plank

1. Place your hands on the floor, under your shoulder blades, and stretch your legs out behind you. Point your toes and let your feet lie on the floor.
2. Activate your core muscles, straighten your arms and draw your belly in towards your spine. Keep your bottom flat and your body super-straight. Hold the position for 10 seconds.

29 Bridging

1. Lie on your back and bend your knees, so your feet are flat on the floor. Arms should be by your side.
2. Suck in your tummy and then lift your bottom off the floor. Lift your pelvis as high off the floor as you can manage until your back is straight. Hold the position for 2 seconds, then release back down.

Getting fit: 3 bridges.
Fighting fit: 5 bridges.
Super-fit: 8 bridges.

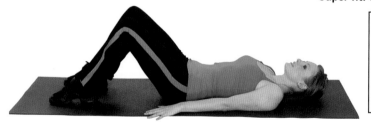

> **PRO TIP:** The bridge is an excellent move for toning your hamstrings and your bottom. To give yourself an extra boost, clench your buttock muscles at the top of the pose, and make sure you really suck in your tummy muscles.

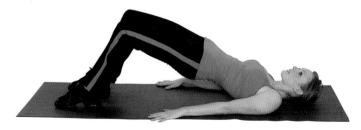

30 Tricep dips

1. Sit on the floor with your legs bent in front of you and your arms behind you.
2. Engage your tricep muscles and push your buttocks and pelvis up towards the ceiling.
3. Lower yourself down and repeat.

Getting fit: 5 reps.
Fighting fit: 8 reps.
Super-fit: 10 reps.

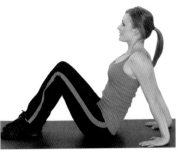

PRO TIP: For a bit of variety, do your tricep dips on the edge of a chair. Place your palms on the edge the seat, and lower yourself up and down, from mid-air to chair-level. But stay away from chairs on wheels, which could slide away as you work out!

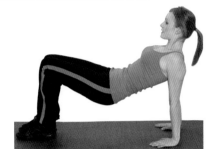

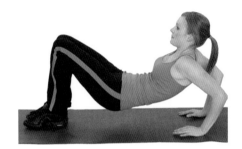

31 Arch-ups

1. Lie on the floor face down, with your feet shoulder-width apart and toes on the mat.
2. Bring your hands to the side of your head and slowly lift your head and shoulders off the floor. This is great for strengthening your back.

Getting fit: 3 reps.
Fighting fit: 5 reps.
Super-fit: 8 reps.

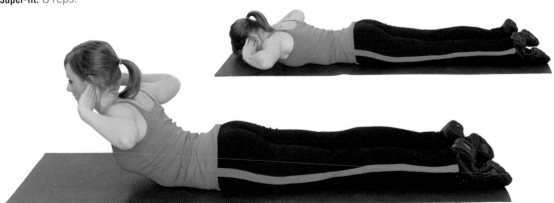

3

The Hip Hop Workout

Hip Hop culture emerged from the ghettos of New York's Bronx district during the turbulent 1970s and 80s. At a time when America's rich were getting richer and poor were getting poorer, dispossessed people used records, microphones and other urban scraps to create an intense sound, driven by a strong beat and pulsating rhythm.

"If you've never tried fast-paced dance before, give Hip Hop a go. You might find it tough at first, but it's an exciting dance style and will help you unleash your inner superstar."

Hip Hop dance grew in response to the fast-paced nature of the music, and today it has evolved into a dance form that's popular on a global scale. Hip Hop is not about grace – it's about sharp, jerky movements and intensity. Even the names of Hip Hop moves sound tough; while ballet dancers do pointe work and pirouettes, Hip Hop dancers do body rocking, popping, krumping and breakdancing.

Today, Hip Hop dance is everywhere you look. Switch on MTV and you'll be bombarded with images of 50 Cent, Missy Elliott, P. Diddy and Jay-Z doing their thing. These Hip Hop artists have become international superstars, famed as much for their music as they are for their bling-bling lifestyles and billion dollar pay cheques.

But at a grass roots level, Hip Hop dance is still about self-expression. Dancers quickly get hooked on the adrenaline that dance gives them, and young people use it as a form of self-expression.

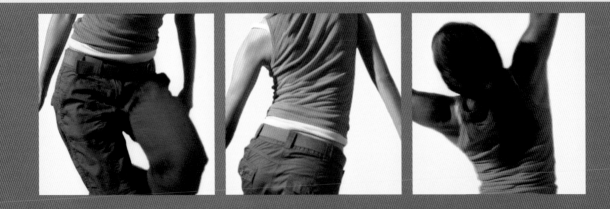

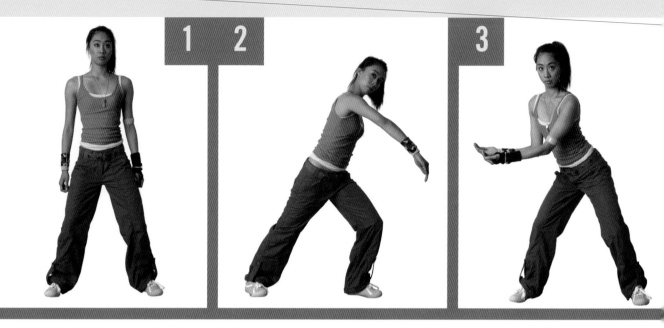

The scoop move

1 Stand with your legs about 1m apart. Bend your knees slightly (in Hip Hop, this is known as 'off-lock') and face the front.

2 Leading with your right arm, bend over to the left and make a 'scoop' shape with your right hand – as if you were capturing an armful of air. Your left knee should stay bent, but your right leg will straighten out as you lean to the left. **(1)** See A note about timing on page 39.

3 Lean over to the right-hand side and with both hands, 'scoop up' the air. **(2)**

4 Using both hands, turn your palms to the floor and 'bounce' the air – first on the left of your body, then on the right. This move is quicker: you should need just one and a half beats to move from left to right. **(3 AND)**

5 Bring your left forearm to your shoulder, keep your palms turned down, and look behind you over your left shoulder. **(4)** Your feet stay stuck to the floor in their initial position until the fourth count of the music, when your left foot steps behind your right foot.

Keep your right arm down at your side and step your left foot behind your right. To maintain some bounce, make sure you keep your heel of your left foot off the floor (weight should be on your tip toes). **(4)**

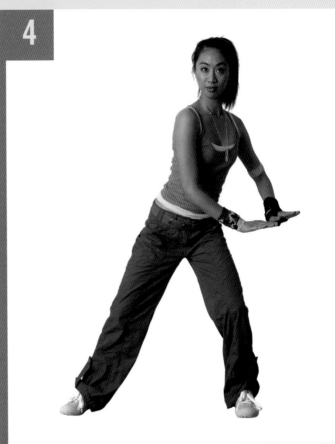

A note about timing

Dance routines are usually choreographed to 8 counts, but because Hip Hop dance is so precise, choreographers sometimes add extra counts, to fit more in. These are known as 'AND counts'. They mean that a routine might be counted: **'1, 2, 3, 4, 5 AND 6, 7 AND 8'**.

In the context of this book, an AND count is a move that happens on a half-beat. It's fast. So rather than taking 3 seconds to dance steps 5 AND 6, you'd only take 2 seconds. The 'AND' bit is squeezed in between the other two moves.

After every move in a routine you'll find a number in brackets. This number is the count that the move should be danced on. If you see **(1)** after an instruction, this is the first move and you should dance it on the first beat of the track. If you see a **(2)**, this should be danced on the second beat. But if you see **(AND)**, this should be danced on a half-beat, before the next numbered count.

At first, it might be easier to give each movement a whole count. But once you've got the hang of the movement, speed things up and introduce the AND counts. This way, you'll be following the lead of Hip Hop pros, and dancing an authentic routine. Good luck!

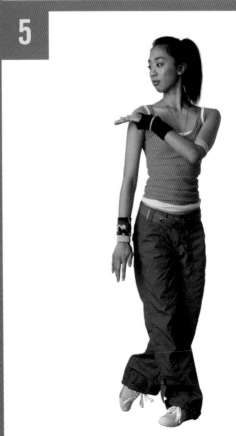

Hip Hop walking

Carrying on from the last position, and the fourth count of the music:

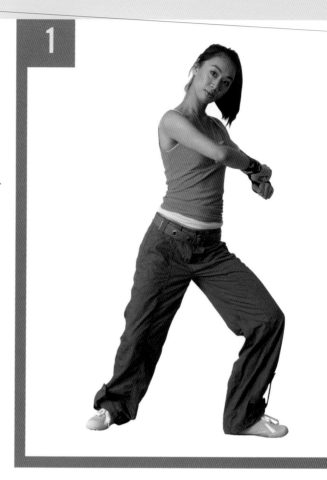

1 Lift your left leg and step forwards on to it (you will be travelling in a slightly diagonal direction). As you step with your left leg, bring your right arm up to chest height. Bend it at the elbow and make a fist with your hands. **(5)**

2 Lift your right leg and 'dig' it into the floor. To do this, lead with your heel and keep your toes off the floor, pointing towards the ceiling. As you dig your foot, bring your left arm up to chest level and bend it at the elbow, fists clenched. Bring your right arm down to your hips and point it away from your body – as if there were a weight leading it towards the back of the room. **(6)**

3 Step your right foot back and bend forwards from your hips. Bring your right arm back to shoulder level (bend it at the elbow) and keep your left arm at the side, leaning towards the back wall. **(7)**

4 Bring your right leg in so it is touching your left leg. Both arms should be temporarily down by your sides. **(AND)**

5 Jump your left foot out. Place the weight on the ball of your foot, bend your knee and lean over to the right. Both arms should be in front of you in a kind of boxed-off shape. **(8)**

❛ Hip Hop keeps my body in great shape. In fact, if I did not dance then my life would be a different story. I have very bad hips and back. But dancing helps keep my posture correct and my muscles strong. And it's a great way to have fun. ❜

2   **3**

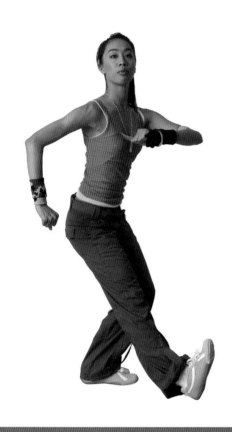

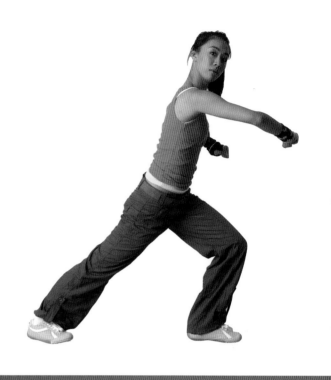

4   **5**

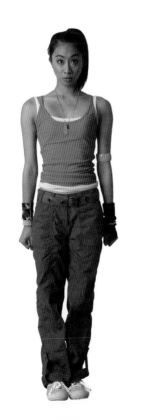

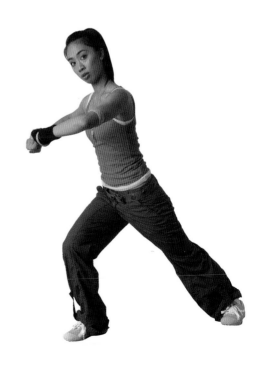

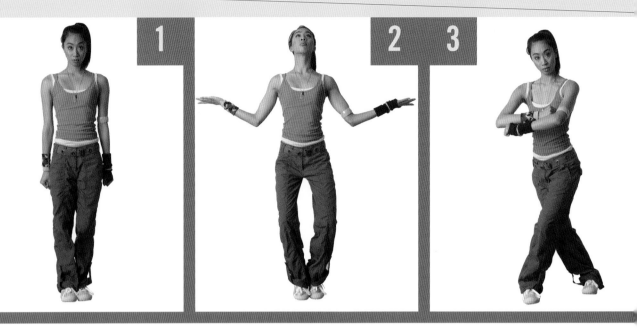

Facing the front

1 Start with your feet together and bring your hands down by your sides. **(1)**

2 Rise up on the balls of both feet and look up. Come down again on an **(AND)** count. Bend your arms at the elbow, so your palms are diagonally facing the ceiling **(2)**. Bring them back down to the side on an **(AND)** count.

3 Cross your left leg in front of your right leg. Clench both fists and bring your arms in front of your body. **(3)**

4 Step your right foot out. Keep both legs bent. As you step your right foot out, scoop your left hand inside the box that your right arm is making, and keep it moving until your left arm is at a 90 degree angle to your right arm.

5 Move your right foot out to the side and straighten both legs so that your feet are about 1m apart. **(4 AND 5)**

6 Step your right foot back in so that your feet are together. Bring your hands down in front of your chest **(AND)**, then take them back out so your lower arm and forearm are at right angles to each other, and look to the ceiling.

7 Bring your hands back to the centre, with your elbows at right angles and closed fists pressed against each other. **(6 AND)**

4

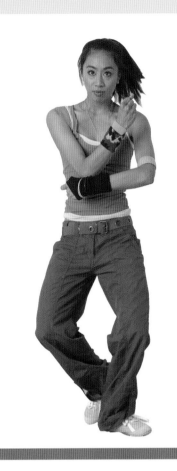

5

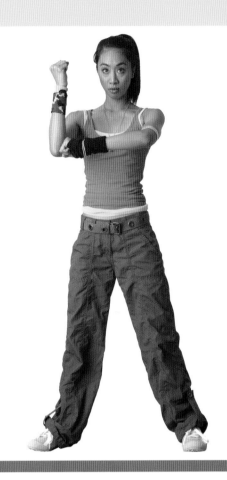

6

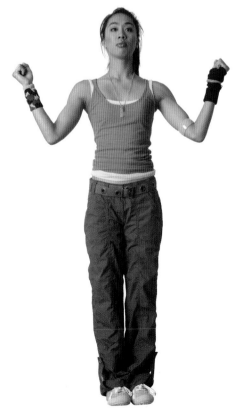

7

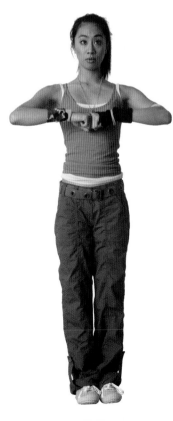

1

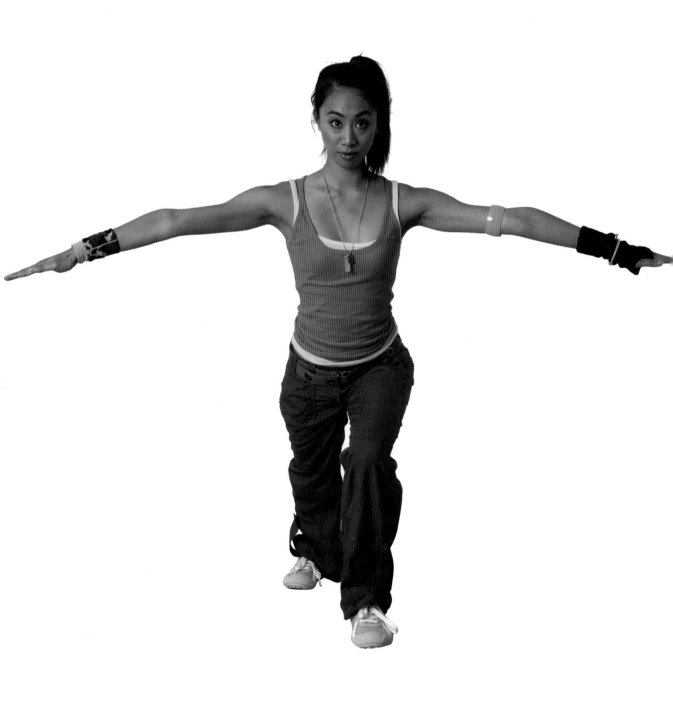

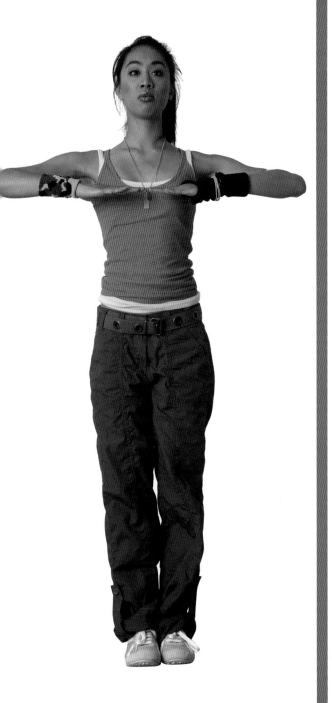

Forward lunge

1 Lunge forwards on your left leg. Keep your knee bent as you move. As you step forwards, lean your torso forwards from your hips. As you lunge, stretch your arms out to the side, like aeroplane wings. **(7)**

2 Then, reversing the previous move, step your left leg back so that your feet are together and both legs are straight. Bring your arms back in. Keep your palms facing downwards and touch your fingertips together. You won't be able to touch all five fingertips, but your index fingers should meet in the middle. **(8)**

Hip Hop is great for:

- Toning your thighs
- Increasing coordination
- Strengthening your ankles
- Loosening your hips
- Toning your waist

2

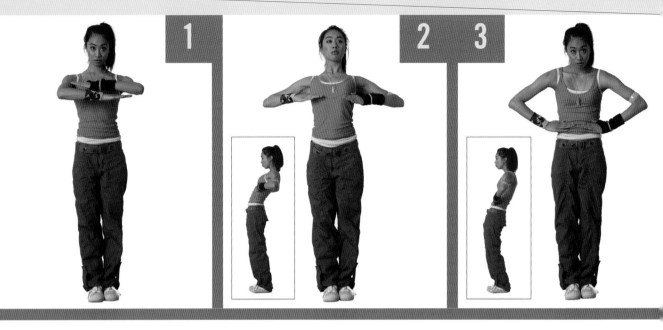

Body roll

1 Stay stationary with your legs together for the first count of the movement. Slide your left arm on top of your right arm. **(AND 1)**

2 Pull your arms back towards your shoulders. Slide them down the side of your body towards the floor. **(1)**

3 As you move your hands, lean your chest backwards and arch your back slightly.

4 Lean your body forwards as you end up with your hands at hip level. Bend your left leg slightly.

5 Lunge your left foot forwards and bend your right leg so that only the ball of your foot is on the floor. Your hands should be facing the floor, at the same level as your left knee. **(2)**

6 Lift your right foot off the floor and flick your heel behind you. Cross your left arm over your right arm. Uncross your arms and circle them around at the side of your head. **(3)**

7 Push your arms back towards floor level. Step your right foot forwards. **(4)**

4

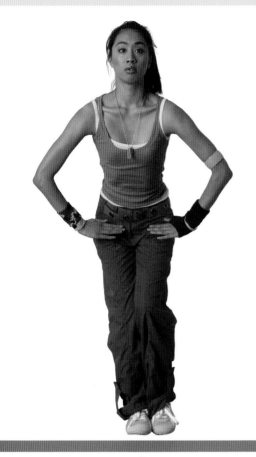

5

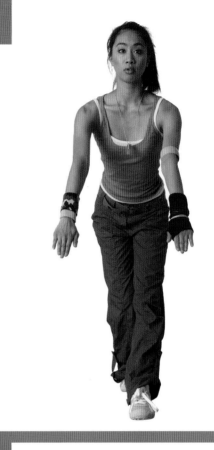

6

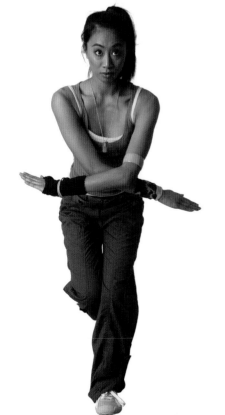

7

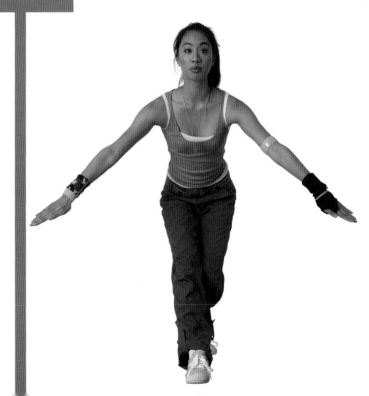

Shoulder roll

1 Take a step to the left with your right leg, moving it in front of your body.

2 As you take the step, touch your right shoulder with your left hand. **(5)** Step out with your right leg, keeping your knee bent. With your left hand, push your right shoulder backwards. Lean over to the right as you push the body away. Your right arm should hang down to the floor – realistically it will sit just above your right knee. **(6)**

❝I have always loved Hip Hop dance. I'm now 46 years old and my body is superb for my age. People tell me I look like I'm in my early 30s. I've got dancing to thank for this – it's kept me fit, healthy and muscular. I can't imagine life without it. ❞

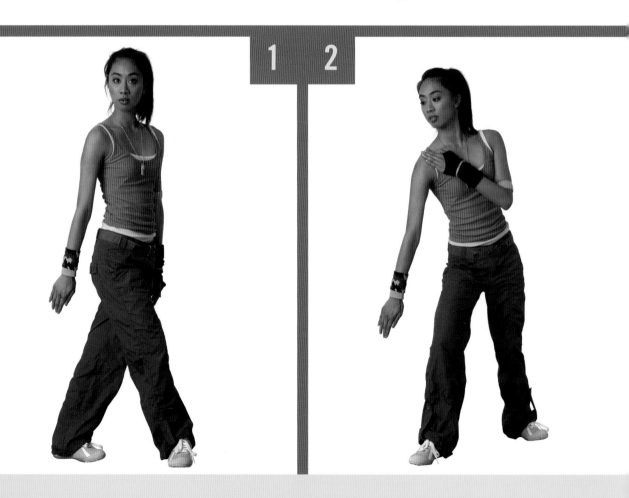

1   2

The turn

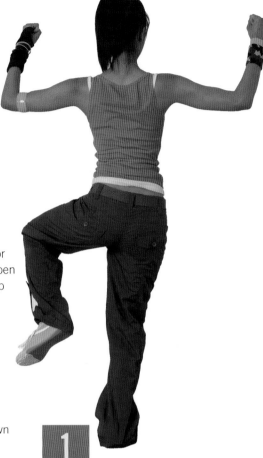

1 To prepare for the turn, let both arms hang down towards the floor and lean forwards, look forward and then cross your arms. **(7)** Open out your arms so that your elbows are bent and at right angles. Lift up your left leg. Your fists should be pointing up towards the ceiling.

2–3 The aim is to spin round 360 degrees in a clockwise direction, keeping the weight on your right leg. **(8)** Put all your energy into spinning. Clench the fists and use your arms as an anchor – the more tension you hold in your arms, the easier it will be for you to spin around.

4 End the turn by lowering your left leg and bringing your arms down to the side of your body.

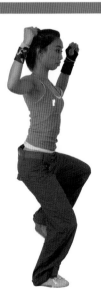

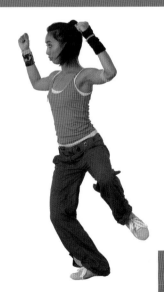

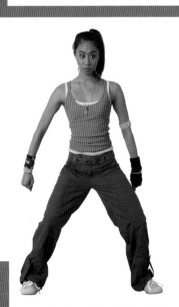

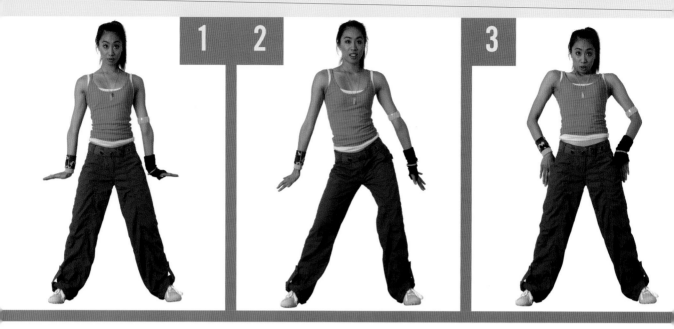

Bounce and shake

1 After the turn, your arms should be by your side. Flex your hands, palms facing the floor. Stand with your legs about 1m apart.

2 Bounce on the spot once. To do this, bend your knees and lift up your feet, elbows and shoulders. Everything should move upwards in one quick move. **(1)** Standing on the spot, shake your knees and bottom rapidly. **(2)**

3—7 From here, go into a body roll. This is similar to the Body Roll on page 46, but this time roll from your hips upwards. Start with your hips, then roll your ribs, your chest, and finally your elbows forwards too. Once your arms are in front of your body with elbows bent, bend your right knee and let your arms lead you over to the right side of your body. **(3 AND 4)**

Pro tip

Don't forget about your arms when executing the body roll. If you relax your arms and let your elbows do the work, the move is a lot easier to pull off.

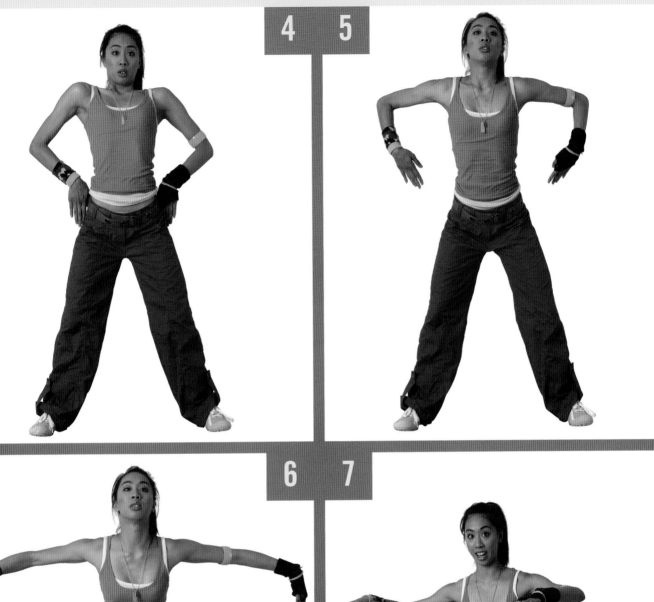

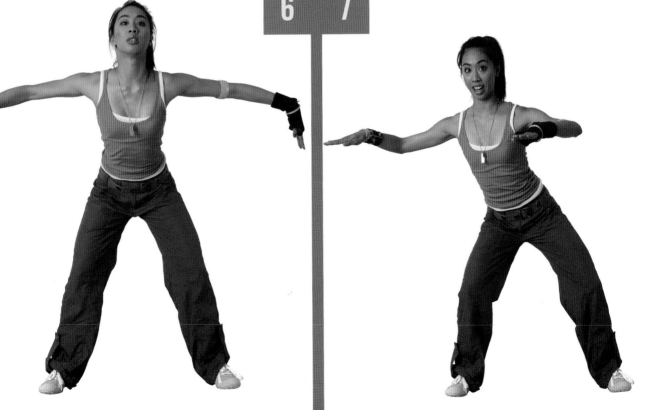

The killer move: tick tock

The tick tock move is featured in many Hip Hop dance routines; it is so called because dancers use their arms and body to mimic the movement of clock hands following each other around in a circle. You start by moving the right hand, and when it hits your chest, you start moving your left hand in the same direction. The whole movement should be completed in nine counts. You can split these counts and the movement in any way you want, but the aim is to have both hands touching on the right-hand side of your body by the time you get to the seventh count of the routine.

The tick tock is a great way to add definition and power to a routine. Follow the instructions below, moving your arms in a graceful, continuous motion. Once you've got the hang of it, tense your upper body and make every movement more mechanical. This will give the move impact and stance, and help you release your inner Hip Hop diva.

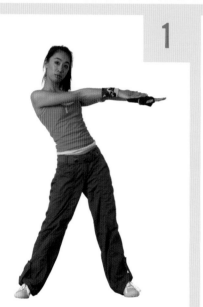 **1**

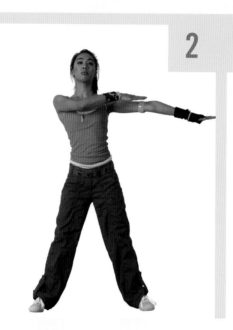 **2** **3**

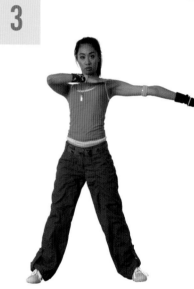

You've got nine counts to complete this move, so make each movement well defined and flex your hands at the end of the motion. Picking up from the end of the last move, the first count will be 3:

1—3 Move your right hand up to the top of your left arm, as if you were pulling your sleeve up. **(3 AND 4)**

4 Move your right arm across your chest. When you are halfway across your chest, bend your left arm and bring your left hand towards your right hand – so your fingertips are almost touching. **(AND 5)**

5—6 Continue the motion with both hands. Both hands should now be moving towards the right with your right hand leading, as if you were pushing the sleeve down on your right arm. **(AND 6)**

7 When both hands have finished moving, they should be touching and be on the right-hand side of your body, with your palms flexed at an angle. **(AND 7)**

4

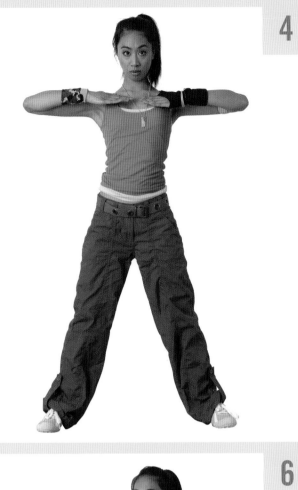

5

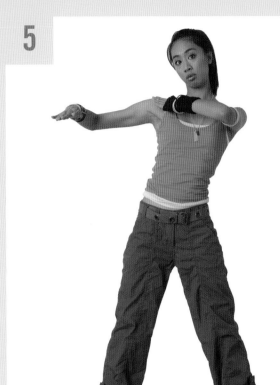

6

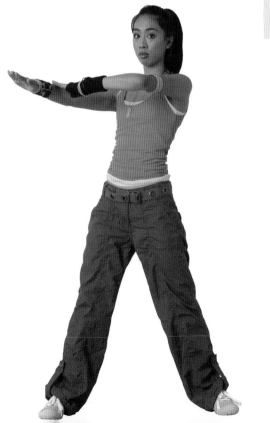

7

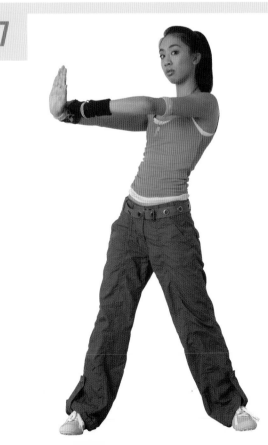

The final pose

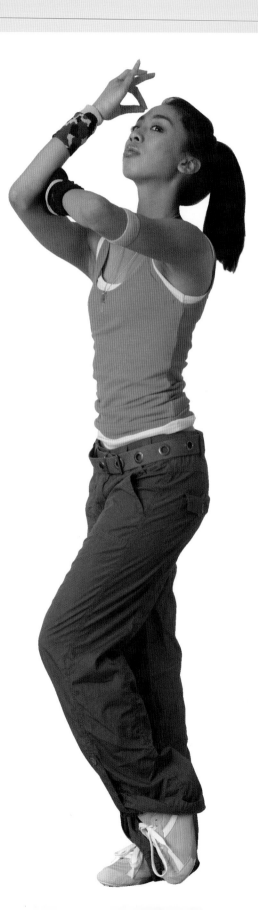

You've got just two counts of the routine to go! To get into your final position:

1 Step your left foot in so that both feet are touching. Bend your left knee so that only the ball of your foot is on the floor.

2 Bend your right arm at the elbow and reach up to touch your head – imagine you are grabbing the brim of a cap **(all these actions happen on the AND count).**

3 Bend your left arm so that your hand is touching the inside of your right forearm.

4 Pull the visor down and look to the floor. This is your final pose and you have finished the Hip Hop routine. **(8)**

To repeat:
Step to your left on your left foot, and walk around in a circular motion, making sure you are back facing the front by the eighth count of the music. Then start the routine again from the beginning, and keep going until the end of the track. Repeat as many times as necessary – this will give you a proper cardio boost and help you maximize the benefits of your workout.

Get creative with your posing!

Switch on MTV and you won't catch Missy Elliott posing in exactly the same way as Beyoncé or Christina. Every Hip Hop diva worth her salt has her own particular stance and way of dancing.

So once you've mastered the final pose suggested here, why not try inventing your own? You can crouch down, lunge forwards, jump into mid-air – whatever you want. Hip Hop dance is a great way to express what's buried deep inside you, so feel free to adapt the moves in this routine as you see fit. The more attitude, the better, so let loose and get posing!

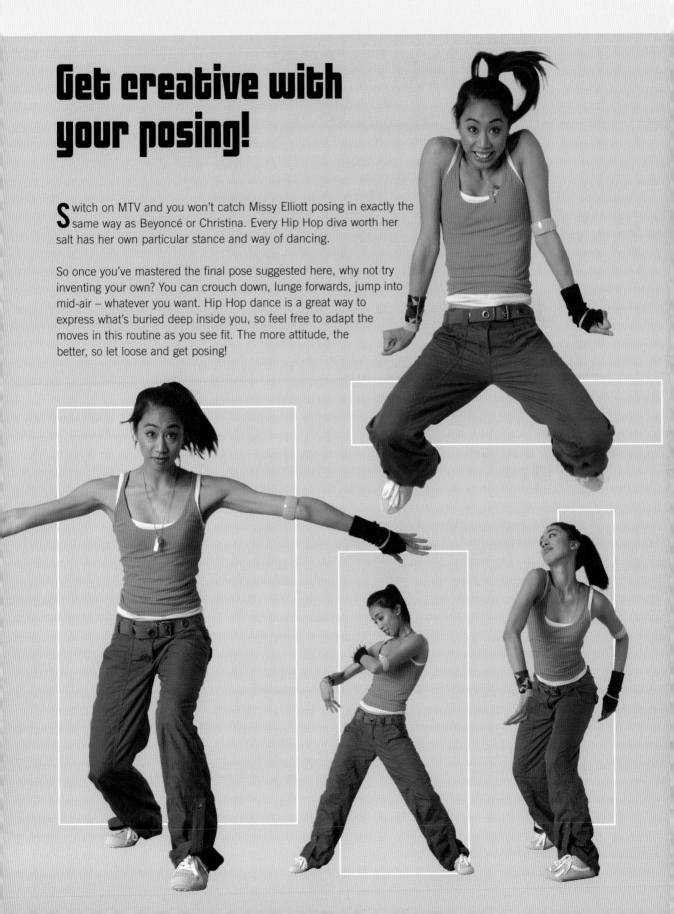

Choosing your music and workout level

This routine can be danced to a fast track or a slow track – it's really up to you which music you choose. The crucial thing to bear in mind is your fitness level: if you're new to exercise and Hip Hop dance in particular, you shouldn't dance to a super-fast beat in your first session. It will exhaust and confuse you far more than is necessary.

To help you pick the right track for your fitness level, below are three playlists. While you're building your confidence and aerobic stamina, work with a song from the first list. When you're feeling stronger, up the pace a notch and choose a track from the second list. And when you're super-strong and dancing like the girls on MTV, pick a fast track from the third list and go for it!

In every case the routine is the same, so make sure you've mastered the moves before you pump up the volume and start working out.

Hip Hop playlists

**GETTING FIT
(slowest tempo)**

1. Missy Elliott
   'I Can't Stand the Rain'
2. Faith Evans
   'Mesmerized'
3. Salt 'N' Pepa
   'Shoop'
4. Dru Hill
   'How Deep is Your Love?'
5. Notorious B.I.G.
   'One More Chance'

**FIGHTING FIT
(medium tempo)**

1. Jill Scott
   'Gimme'
2. Busta Rhymes
   'Touch It'
3. Petey Pablo featuring
   Rasheeda
   'Vibrate'
4. Ying Yang Twins
   'Shake'
5. Mary J. Blige featuring
   Will Smith
   'Got To Be Real'

**SUPER-FIT
(up-tempo)**

1. Missy Elliott
   'Lose Control'
2. Christina Aguilera and Missy
   Elliott 'Car Wash'
3. Field Mob featuring
   Ciara
   'So What'
4. Nelly Furtado featuring
   Timbaland
   'Promiscuous'
5. Magoo and Timbaland
   'Drop'

Case study

Zievrina Wilson, 28, a teacher from south-west London, dropped two dress sizes through dancing Hip Hop in her living room. She now teaches street dance classes for young people in her spare time.

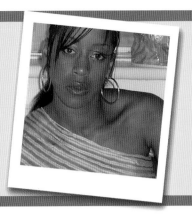

'I took my first Hip Hop class when I was a teenager. My mum was a drama teacher and she was running a street dance workshop for some of her students. I went along to her class one day and I had a great time. The routine we learned was cool – it was full of funky steps and was heaps more fun than the ballet routines I'd learned as a child, and I left the class with a massive smile on my face!

'Since then, I've become a complete Hip Hop dance addict. I'm a performing arts teacher and although I love my job, a typical day at college can leave me stressed out. To help me relax, the first thing I do when I get home is turn my stereo up loud and do some Hip Hop dancing. I'll usually dance to Missy Elliott, Busta Rhymes or P. Diddy.

'My favourite street dance song of all time is 'Ain't No Stoppin' Us,' from the 80s film *Breakdance*. I don't follow a set routine, I just listen to the beat of the music and throw my body around. Dance is like a drug to me. It releases so many feel-good hormones that I feel happier the instant I start moving.

'Hip Hop gives me an all-over workout and when I sweat, I feel like I'm sweating the pounds away.'

'Dance is also having an amazing effect on my body. Since I upped the frequency of my dancing to three times per week, for two hours each time, I've found it easier to tone up. I've dropped two dress sizes – I used to be a size 12, but now I'm an 8. My thighs are much more toned and I've gained stronger stomach and buttock muscles. I can wear little T-shirts and skinny jeans because my body is firmer. My bikini looked fantastic this summer! My husband is impressed with my slender new figure, but what he really loves is the body confidence that comes with it. I used to dislike my hips and thighs but now when I look in the mirror I see a leaner physique than before and I love it!

'Hip Hop gives me an all-over workout and when I sweat, I feel like I'm sweating the pounds away. If you're reading this book and wondering if Hip Hop dance is for you, I challenge you to turn the music up loud and give it a go. Hip Hop dance allows you to shake your body in a way that is fun and accessible to everyone. You don't need dance experience and you don't need to know loads about Hip Hop culture. Just put some trainers on, clear a space in your living room and go for it. My bet is that you'll love it, and you'll soon be flaunting your moves in public like a real dancing queen!'

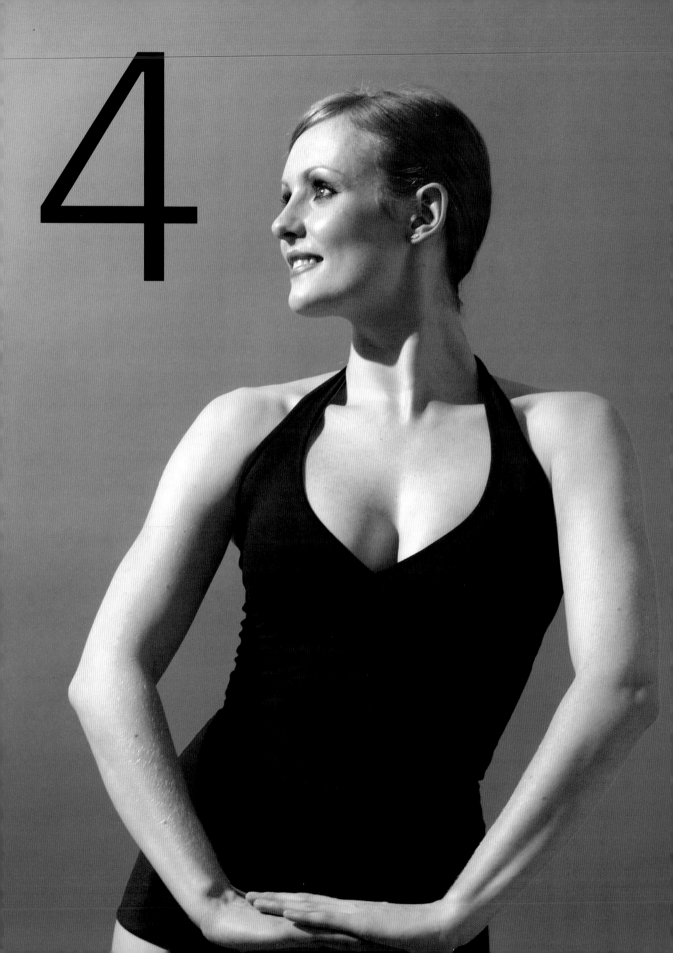

4

The Broadway Workout

Midtown Manhattan has been buzzing with the glamour, glitz and all-round fabulousness of showbusiness since 1886, when a play called *The Black Crook* took Broadway by storm. Featuring a chorus of a hundred high-kicking female ballerinas, the show took over a million pounds at the box office and heralded the birth of a new theatrical form: the musical.

Since then, the streets of Broadway – and those in other cities across the globe – have been awash with jaw-dropping musical theatre productions that have stunned audiences and kept them begging for more. 'Broadway dance' is a catch-all phrase, and in this book it's used to refer to shows that incorporate elements of jazz, tap, ballet and contemporary dance. In reality, every musical in gives audiences something different. Shows such as *Fame* and *Footloose* are fast-paced and energetic, while the newer shows often transport audiences to a fantasy land.

If there's one thing that unites all Broadway and West End shows it's the honest enthusiasm and passion that underscores every movement. Broadway dance is not about being cool or saving face; it's about storytelling and entertaining. So slick on some lip gloss and get your jazz hands at the ready. It's time to try some Broadway dance…

> ❛ **Broadway can be fast paced and energetic or controlled and sexy and it is always about storytelling and entertaining.** ❜

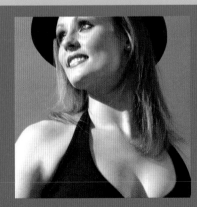 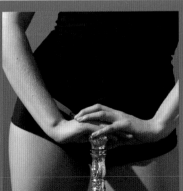 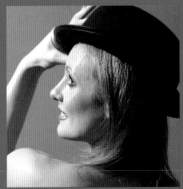

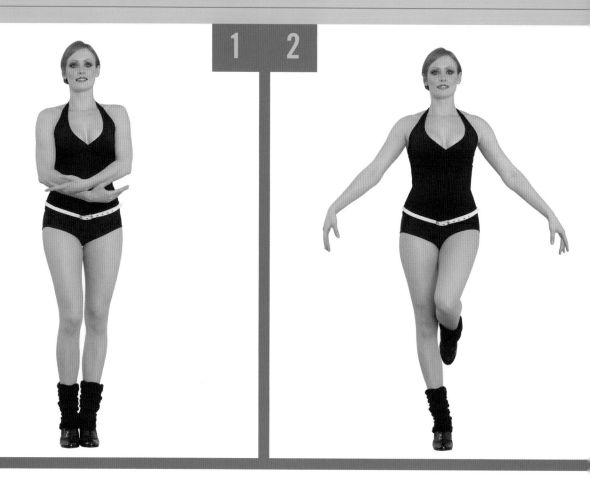

Building the drama

1—4 Starting with your left foot and alternating your feet, gently tap 16 times on the spot. At the same time, stretch your arms out sideways and slowly move them up until they cross over your head and your right hand is touching your left elbow **(this should take eight counts)**.

5—6 Slowly unfurl your arms and bring them back to the starting position at the front of your body **(this should also take eight counts)**.

Pro tip

Use the opening bars of the music as a time to focus your energies and slip into 'performance mode'. As leading dance teachers will tell you, what you do with your eyes and face is just as important as what you do with your body when you're on a Broadway stage. So, imagine you are playing to a packed house on 42nd Street, and perform!

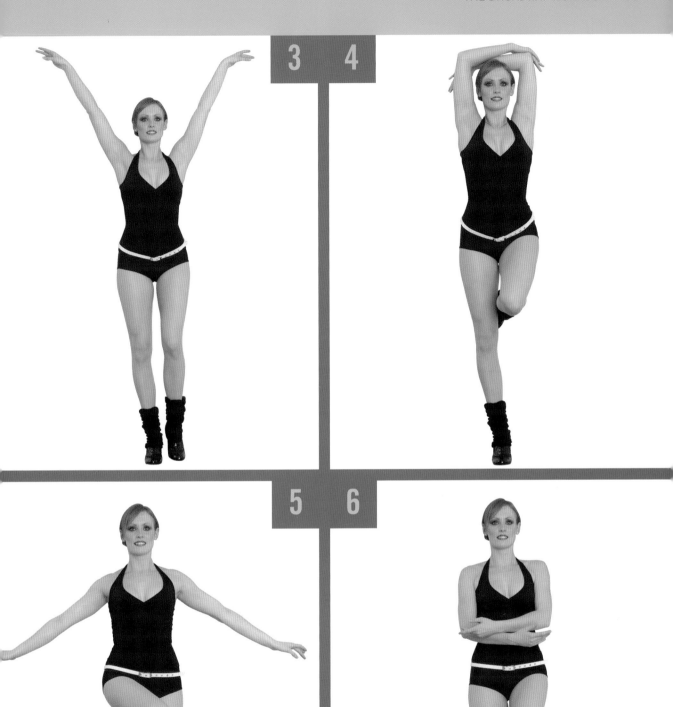

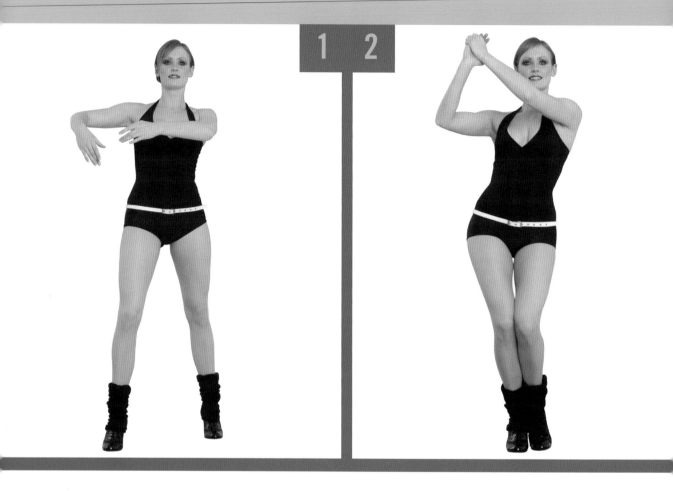

Overhead claps

1 Step forwards on your right leg at a diagonal of 30 degrees. Keep your head facing the front.

2 Step your left foot forwards to meet your right foot. As you do this, clap overhead – once on the right, once on the left.

3 Then step your right foot back at a diagonal of 30 degrees – so it's returning to the same place that it came from. Keep your head facing the front.

4 Then step your left foot in so it is touching your right foot. Clap twice more as you step backwards, except this time lean forwards from your hip and clap just above your knees.

3 **4**

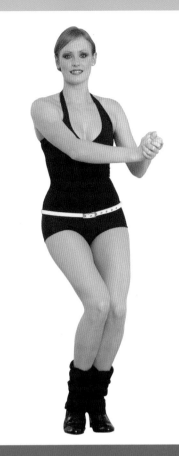

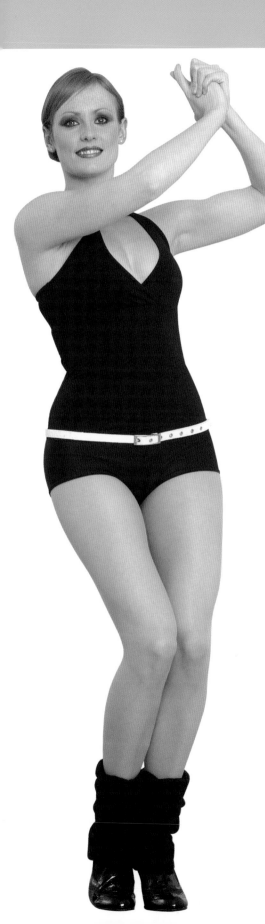

Broadway dance is good for:

- Strengthening the lower back
- Tightening the core muscles and abs
- Increasing balance and poise
- Correcting postural problems

Side show

1 Step to the side on your right leg and lift your left leg up, so that your left foot is next to your right knee. If you can balance, try to rise up on to the ball of your right foot, so that all the weight is in your toes. Bend your right arm at the elbow, point it to the right side of the room and splay your fingers as wide as they can go. Bend your left arm at the elbow and place your hand on your left hip. Splay the fingers of your left hand, and look forwards.

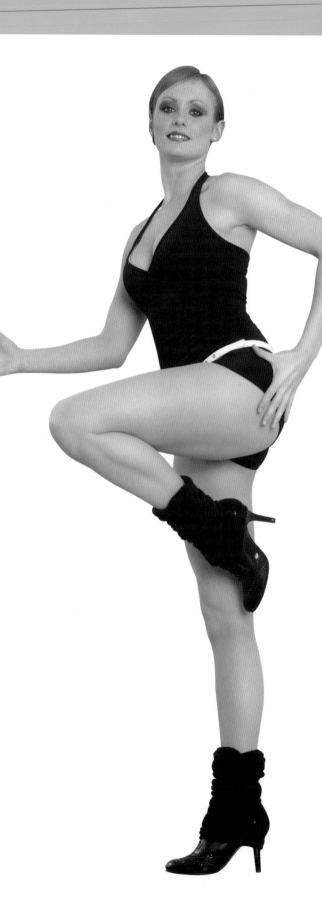

Pro tip

The moves in this section are as much about posing and performing as they are about dancing.

To help you get the hang of the movements, each move has been broken down into a series of actions. Start off by practising different actions in isolation, and then put them together once you've got the hang of it.

Travelling step

1 Bring your left foot down to the floor and step on to it. Travelling in a diagonal direction, stretch your right foot out and point your toe. Keep your left arm touching your waist. Stretch your right arm out and place it elegantly down by your side. Flex your hand and fix your gaze so that you are looking down at your right hand.

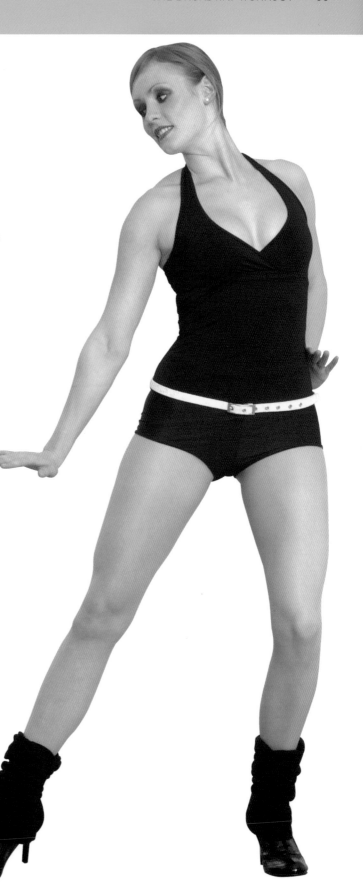

'Broadway dance has boosted my body confidence 100% and improved my social life too. I used to be quite shy but these days I'm the first on the dance floor at parties, and I use my Broadway moves to flirt with men. It's my secret pulling trick and it works every time!'

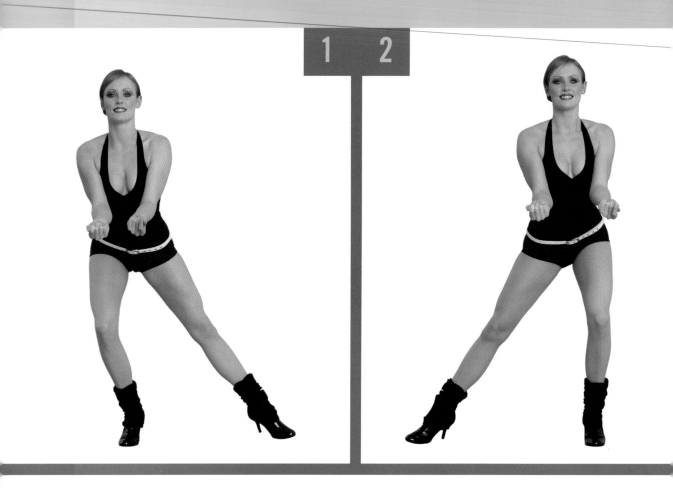

Click steps

1 Lift your right foot off the floor and take two steps towards the left side of the room, on a diagonal of 30 degrees. At the end of the second step, point the toes of your left foot. Keep your body low as you move, and once you've completed your second step to the left, flick your wrists forwards and click your fingers once, directly in front of you.

2 Repeat on the other side. Start with your left leg, step towards the right side of the room on a diagonal of 30 degrees. At the end of the second step, point the toes of your right foot. Repeat the finger click once you've travelled to the right.

Stepping back

1 Facing the front, step back on your right foot, then step back on your left foot. As you move, turn towards the left side of the room, so you end up facing the back. Step forwards on your left foot. Punch your right arm into the air, splaying your fingers.

2 Keep your legs apart and bend both knees. Flick your right hip out, as if you were sitting on a chair. As you do this, your left heel will come off the floor and your weight will transfer to your right leg. As you flick your hip out to the right, bring your right arm down to chest height and point your forearm out to the right. Keep energy in your arm and splay your fingers. At the same time, bring your left arm up to shoulder height. Bend it at the elbow and touch your thumb and index finger together. Splay the rest of your fingers and touch the left side of your head – as if you were realigning a bowler hat.

Pro tip

Many moves in this routine are inspired by the work of Bob Fosse, an American choreographer born in 1927, who created routines for the original Broadway productions of *Chicago*, *Cabaret* and *Sweet Charity*. Splayed fingers and hunched shoulders won't feel right the first time you do them, but they are typical of the Fosse style and look super-slick on stage. To maximize your chances of getting it right, forget big gestures and focus instead on really controlling your movements. This routine doesn't require mid-air jumps and leaps across the stage – it just needs energy, precision and showbiz flair.

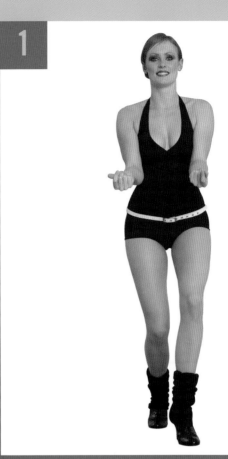

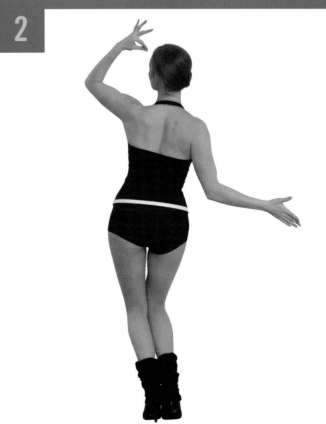

Arm and leg flick

1 Standing on the spot, transfer the weight on to your left leg and flick your left hip out. Your right heel will come off the floor and your knee should be bent; only the ball of your foot is on the floor. Bend both your arms at the elbow. Keeping them behind you, flick both your arms out to the left side of your body. Splay your fingers, and move them to the left at exactly the same time that you pop your hip to the left. Your right palm should be visible; your left palm should be facing the back of the room.

2 Reverse the previous move: transfer the weight on to your right leg and flick your right hip out. Your left heel will come off the floor and your knee should be bent; only the ball of your foot is on the floor. Flick your arms the other way so they are now pointing out to the right. Reverse your palms, so that now your left palm is visible and your right palm is facing the back of the room.

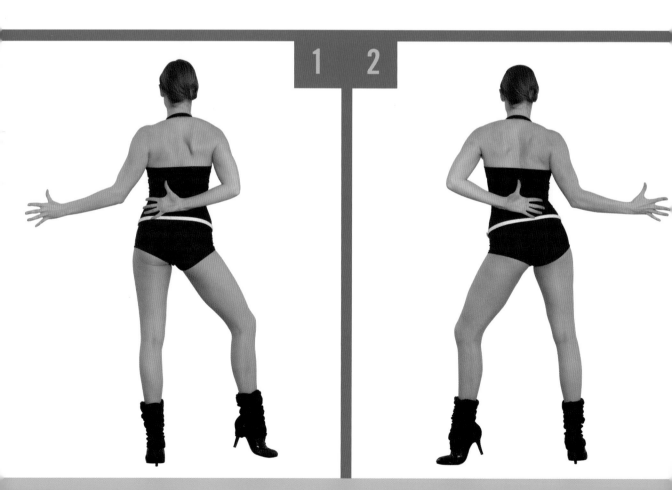

Step and turn

1 Start this move while you are still facing the back of the room. Slowly lower your arms to the side. Transfer the weight on to your right foot and lift your left leg up. Spin round on your right foot and face the front. Step your left foot to the side and turn your body as you walk. Step on to your right foot and transfer the weight. Lift your left leg and bring your knee up so it is touching the right knee. Bend your left arm, and place it on your hip with your fingers facing the floor.

As your left leg is lifting, slide your left arm up your body until it reaches the side of your chest. At the same time, plunge your right hand down towards the floor and flex your hand when it is fully outstretched. Look to the floor and tilt your body over to the right.

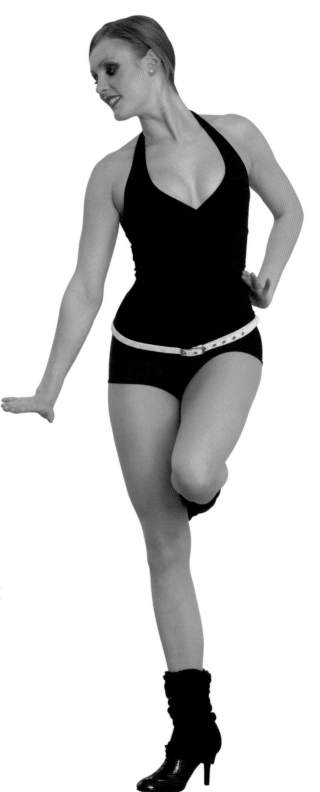

❝I love the pizazz of Broadway dance and the feeling of saying to the world "look at me, here I am, aren't I fabulous!" The adrenaline keeps me going, and I never want to stop – no matter how physically exhausted I might be. I love it! ❞

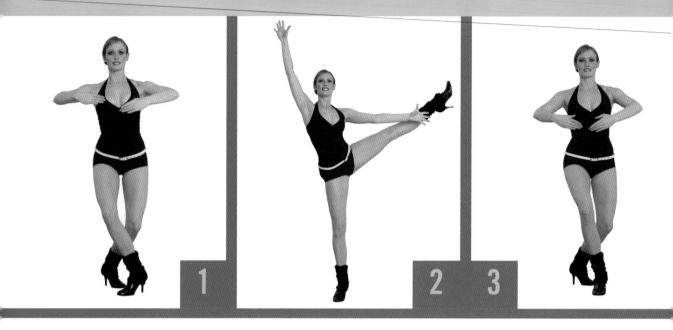

Step and kick

1 Cross your right leg in front of your left leg. Bend your arms at the elbow and bring your fingertips so they are almost touching in front of your chest.

2 Keeping the weight on your right leg, lift your left leg and kick it out to the side. Raise your right arm as you do this, and stand tall.

3 Bring your left leg back down and step your left foot behind your right leg. Bring your arms back to chest level, so that your fingertips are almost touching in front of your body.

4 Bring your right hand up to touch your head. Your forefinger and thumb should be touching and your other three fingers should be splayed as wide as possible. Bring your left elbow in to touch your left hip, and extend your forearm out away from the body. Point your fingers.

5 Keeping both feet on the floor, spin on the spot in an anticlockwise direction, so you end up turning 360 degrees.

6 Keeping your left arm in the same position, raise your right hand to the bowler hat position.

Pro tip

Who is watching you when you step-kick your way across the room? There might not be anyone else there, but imagine you're performing to a particular kind of audience and your moves will suddenly have more meaning. Think like an actor. Are you kicking agressively? Happily? Dance with a different attitude each time you do this workout and give your mind a workout too!

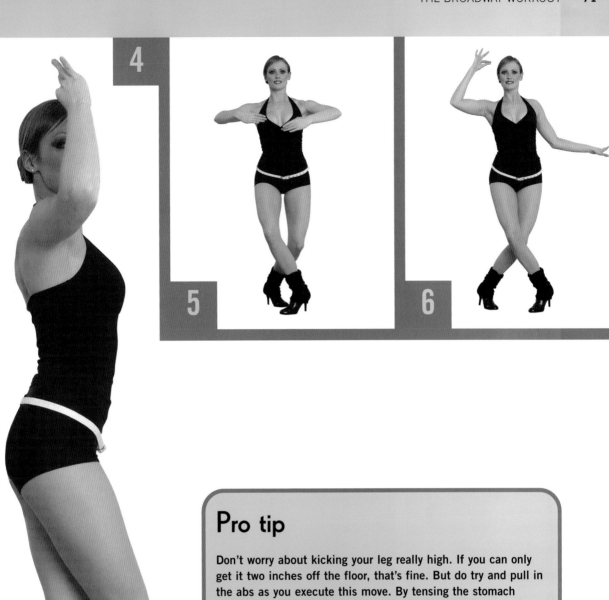

Pro tip

Don't worry about kicking your leg really high. If you can only get it two inches off the floor, that's fine. But do try and pull in the abs as you execute this move. By tensing the stomach muscles, you are grounding your body and making the most of your core strength; this will help you stand tall, and over time, it will make it easier for you to raise the leg a bit higher. Point the toes, too, to really give yourself a showgirl's finesse!

The killer move: the pirouette

To increase the showbiz fabulousness of your routine, replace the mini turn after the leg kick with a pirouette.

But don't panic if you can't get it right straight away – the pirouette is a tricky move to master and your success with it will depend on your balance, coordination and flexibility – and these will differ from day to day.

One way to make this move a bit easier is to split it into four parts. Practise the move by turning just a quarter of the way around the circle. Rather than spinning 360 degrees on your first go, try moving just 90 degrees to the right. Done this way, it should take you four turns to make it back to the centre. It might sound laborious, but each of these mini pirouettes will help you to build your confidence for the main turn. So don't be afraid – practise your turns over and over, and soon you'll be knocking them dead on the dancefloor with a perfect pirouette – take it from a girl who used to have two left feet and now can't stop flaunting the killer moves!

1 Face the front with your legs together, so both your feet are parallel. Bring both arms in front of you, at about chest height, and square them off as if you were holding a beach ball.

2 Step your left foot forwards and bend your knee. Your weight should be on this leg. Slightly bend your right leg and lift your right heel – only the ball of your right foot should be on the floor. As you begin the turn, move your left arm back slightly. Then, once you are turning, bring your left arm back in and use it to power your turn. Strategic arm movements really will help you to get round in one go.

3 Spin around to the right, turning through 360 degrees. To do this, keep your left leg on the floor and raise your right leg so your foot is touching your left knee. Done correctly, you'll be making a triangular shape with your right leg, except the triangle will be pointing to the front, not the side (as you sometimes see in ballet pirouettes).

4 Land with your right foot in front of you – this will leave you in the perfect position to carry on with the next step of the routine.

Pro tip

To help you land in the same place after you turn, focus on a particular spot in front of you for the duration of this move. 'Spotting', as dance teachers call it, will stop you veering off to the left or right. It doesn't matter what you focus on – a picture on the wall would be fine. But your gaze should be fixed on a stationary object – keep your eyes on it for as long as possible before you turn.

1   2

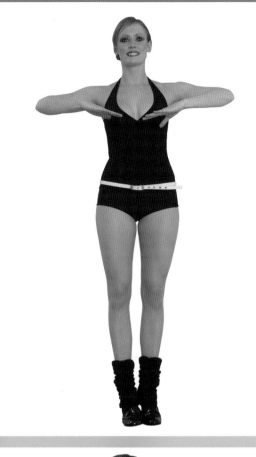 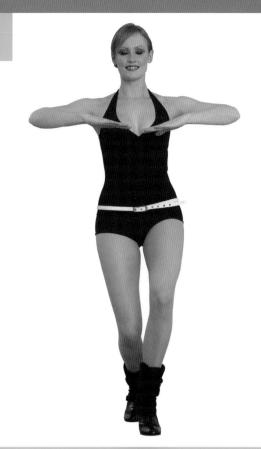

3   4

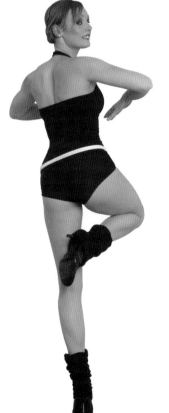 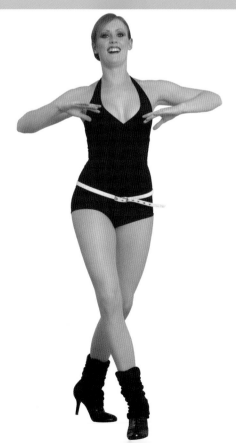

Leg lift

Pro tip

This leg-lift is a classic Broadway move, but if you can only get your right foot a couple of inches off the ground, don't worry. Professional dancers are always taught to perform with their faces as much as with their feet – the idea being that if they dazzle audiences with a megawatt smile, no one will notice if the feet go wrong. Plus, as your flexibility and balance increase, you'll be able to move the leg ever higher, which will give you something to aim for.

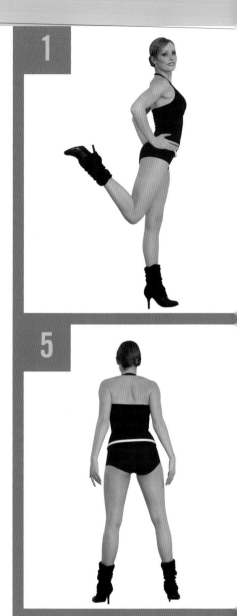

1 Pivot on your heels so you are facing your right side of the room. Place both hands on your hips and flick your right heel up and back behind you.

2 Bring your right leg down and step it out so that you turn towards the back of the room, but keep your heel of your right foot off the floor. Weight is in your left leg, which is straight. Splay the fingers of your right hand.

3 Transfer your weight on to your right foot and step your left foot forwards. As you do this, bring your right arm forwards and down. Flex your hand.

4 Lift your right leg and bring your right foot up to touch your inner thigh. Your right thigh should be parallel to the floor.

5 Lower your right leg, relax your hands and pivot on your heels so that you are facing the back of the room.

6 Spin round 180 degrees on your right foot, so you end up facing the front. Step your right foot in front of your left and bring your arms together in front of your chest, so your fingertips are almost touching.

7 Kick out with your left leg and bring your left arm out to shoulder height in front of your left leg. Raise your right arm up into the air. Splay your fingers and smile!

8 Bring your left leg back down and step it in front of your right leg. Keep your arms extended.

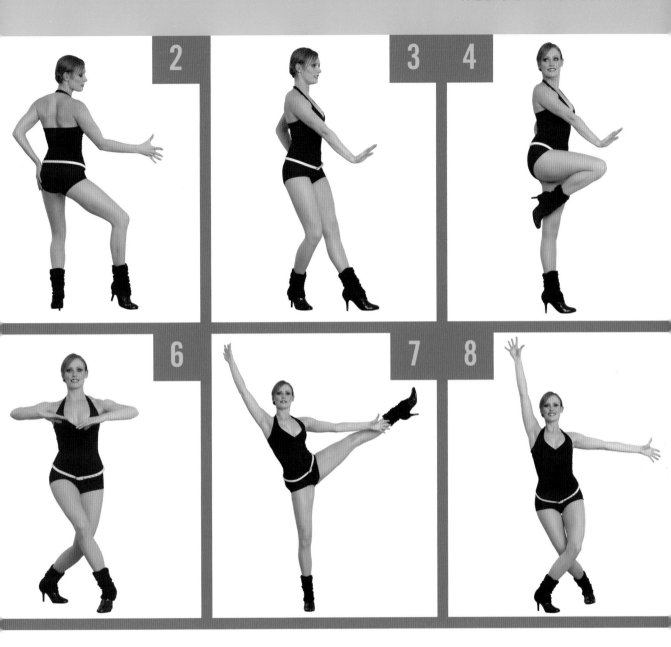

Body flick

1 Step your right foot out and straighten your leg. Open your arms out to make a square shape. Look to the floor.

2 Pop your right hip out and bend your right knee. As you do this, bring your hands in towards your thighs and start to move them up your thighs.

3 Straighten your right knee and level your hips up. Your hands should still be moving up your body, towards your chest.

4 Step your right foot in and straighten both legs. Your hands should be moving towards your head.

5 When your hands reach shoulder height, lift your right foot off the floor and flick your heel back behind you.

6 Finally, stretch your arms above your head and flick your fingers towards the sky. Smile and pose – you have just completed the Broadway workout!

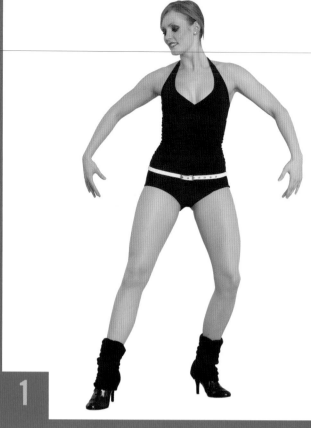

1

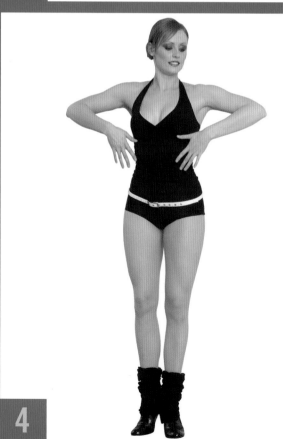

4

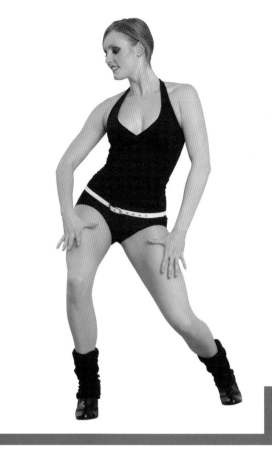

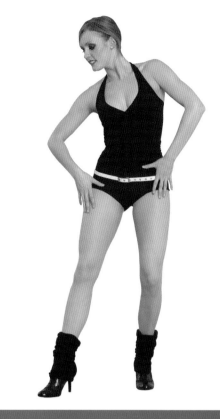

2 3

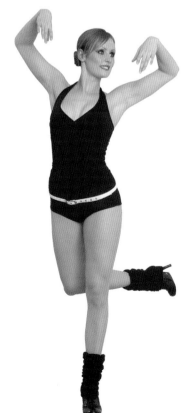

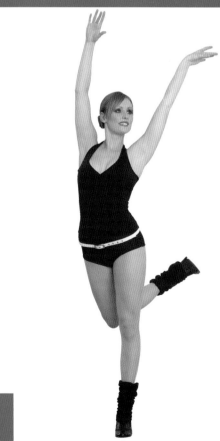

5 6

Choosing your music and workout level

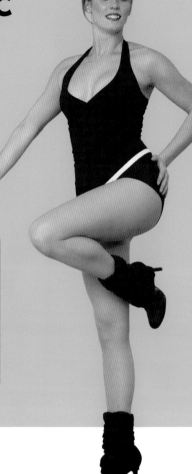

This routine can be danced to a fast or slow beat – the pace you choose depends on your fitness level. Of course, you don't have to choose a track from a musical, but a dramatic song will help you unleash your Broadway spirit. Why not try one of the songs from the playlists below?

Pro tip

In any Broadway or West End show you're bound to see showgirls leaping across the stage while singers use words to tell the story. Dance and drama are one and the same thing in musical theatre, so embrace the super-charged nature of these songs and get dancing!

Broadway playlists

GETTING FIT (level 1)

Ease yourself into Broadway by dancing to one of these not-too-fast tunes:

1. 'Boogie Shoes' from *Saturday Night Fever*
2. 'Grease Is The Word' from *Grease*
3. 'Overture/All That Jazz' from *Chicago*

FIGHTING FIT (level 2)

Step things up a notch by dancing to these up-tempo numbers:

1. 'Cool' from *West Side Story*
2. 'Crazy' from *Starlight Express*
3. 'Fame' from *Fame*

SUPER-FIT (level 3)

Feel Broadway-fabulous by dancing to these super-fast tracks:

1. 'Footloose' from *Footloose*
2. 'Don't Stop Me Now' from *We Will Rock You*
3. 'Dancing Through Life' from *Wicked*

Case study

Rebecca Dent, 24, from Lancashire, went from waitress to West End star after winning a British TV talent competition. Here she explains how dancing has re-shaped her body – and banished her bad moods – once and for all.

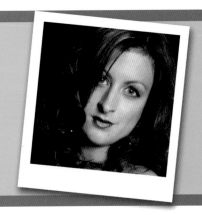

'Before I won Channel 4's Musicality programme in 2004, I was working as a waitress in a local pub. I tried to get to the gym at least once a week but that sometimes didn't happen. My most strenuous exercise came from carrying heavy dishes to tables. I wasn't paranoid about my weight but every time I gained a few pounds, it showed. My body had its fair share of wobbly bits and sometimes I'd catch a glimpse of myself in the mirror and feel a bit depressed.

Then, after several rounds of auditions, I found out I'd won the chance to play Roxie Hart in the London production of *Chicago*. I had just six weeks to master complicated dance routines and morph myself into a leading lady. To say I was scared was an understatement! Thankfully though, the adrenaline got me through and the one-off performance went amazingly well. A week after the show, I auditioned for the part of Annette in *Saturday Night Fever*. Amazingly, I got the job and spent the next 18 months performing eight shows a week to packed houses in theatres across the UK.

'I've lost 10 pounds and have a much flatter stomach than ever before.'

Since dance became a major part of my life I've been a different person. It's true what they say about endorphins being released by exercise – some days I'd go to work in bad mood, but after the first dance number, my heart would be racing and a massive smile would be beaming across my face. My body has changed for the better, too. I don't develop muscle tone very easily and years of pounding the treadmill never got me into great shape. But dance has worked wonders for my arms and legs. My stomach is flatter and I've lost 10 pounds in weight.

Of course, you don't have to dance professionally to feel the benefits. My boyfriend doesn't have great coordination but I've taught him some moves and now he can turn me and lead me across the dance-floor. He hates to admit it but his posture has improved and I know that secretly he enjoys it!

Routines like the one in this chapter can keep you in great shape. This is down to the subtle details of Broadway dancing. Forget big gestures – follow the sultry routine in this book three times per week and you'll soon see positive changes all over your body. You'll also develop greater confidence and better coordination than ever before. If you've got a bit of a showman side to your personality, my tip is to get out there and give dancing a go. You'll be bitten by the bug and you won't be able to stop. I certainly am not going to!'

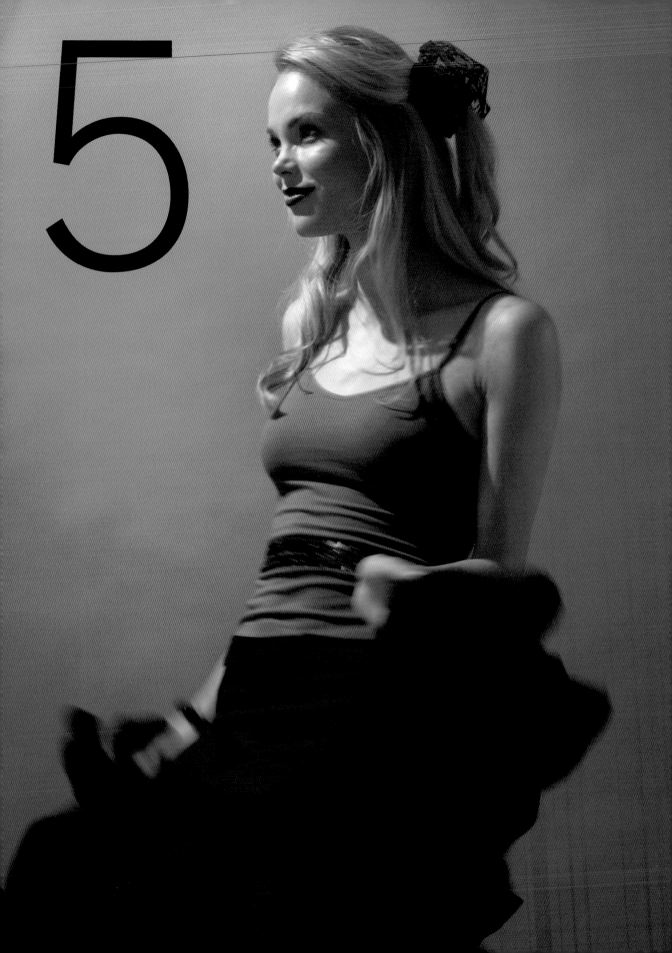

The Latin Workout

I f you like your dance to be exuberant, unpredictable and driven by passion, Latin dance is the style for you. Originating in countries such as Brazil, Argentina and Cuba, Latin dance is an umbrella term used to describe dances such as Salsa, Tango, Mambo, Merengue, Rumba and Capoeira.

Latin dance is popular because it's both beautiful and accessible. The steps are easy to pick up and it can be danced with a huge group of friends in tow, and you don't need to be amazingly coordinated or flexible to glide your way across the dancefloor. Furthermore, if celebrities such as Patsy Palmer (an actress) and Zoë Ball (a DJ) can master the Argentinean Tango on the BBC's *Strictly Come Dancing*, then why on earth can't we give it a go, too?

The routine in this chapter incorporates elements of Salsa, Cha Cha and Tango. It's great for toning the legs and trimming the waist and it will do wonders for your confidence too. The routine will work best if you let your hair down, put on a swirly skirt and let your inhibitions go. Latin dance is about performing with passion – so lose that stiff upper lip and get dancing!

> **Latin dance is beautiful, accessible and easy to pick up. You can dance it with a group of friends or alone and you don't have to be incredibly flexible.**

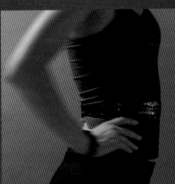
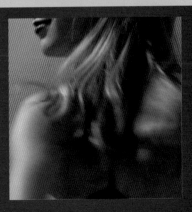

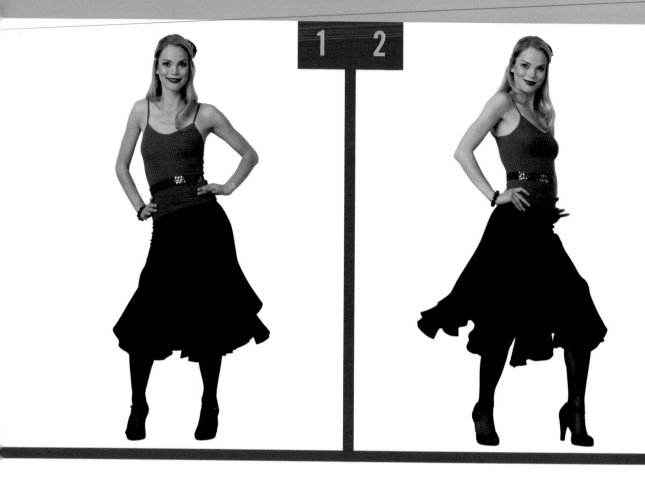

Hip swing

A note on the timing of Latin dance

For this routine, the ideal timing counts are shown in brackets after every move. If you see the number **(1)** after a move, this means the step should be danced on the first count of the music. If you see **(2, 3)**, this means the two steps come on the second and third count of the music, and they follow on directly from each other, with no pause. Try and dance to this tempo, but if you find the moves too fast, halve the speed by adding in another **8** counts to every section. Find a pace that works for you, and enjoy.

1 Stand with your feet hip-width apart. With your arms slightly bent, place your hands loosely on your hips.

2 Gently flick your hips up and out from left to right, keeping the movements as relaxed and fluid as possible. Repeat 10 times.

3 Stand with your feet hip-width apart. With your arms slightly bent, place your hands loosely on your hips.

4 Slowly roll your hips in a full circle, from left to right. To do this, tilt your pelvis forwards and let your hip bones lead your body. Draw five circles to the right, then reverse the motion and draw five circles to the left. This will warm up your hips and leave you ready for the next move.

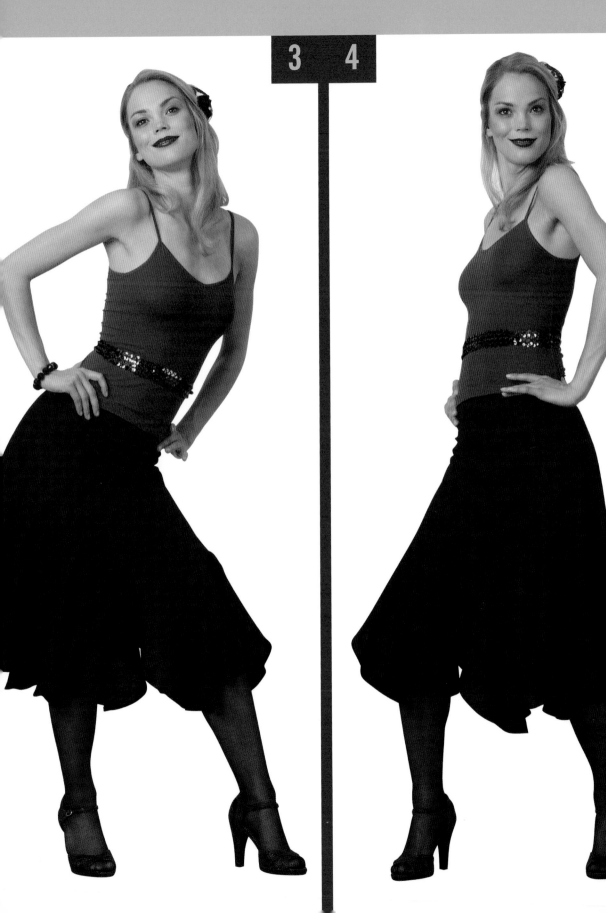

3   4

Salsa step on the right

1 Start with your feet hip-width apart. Step your right foot forwards. Transfer the weight on to the ball of your right foot – your left heel will come off the floor. If you're wearing a skirt, you can take hold of it and swish it around as you're moving **(1)**.

2 Step on to your left foot and take your right foot back – keep moving it past its original position and place it on the floor approximately 0.5m further back than it was at the start **(2)**.

Pro tip

As you move your legs forwards and backwards, your hips will automatically rise and fall. Don't let this put you off! Like Burlesque dance, Latin dance is very hip-driven. So let your body move naturally and embrace the Latino spirit!

‘ Latin dance has definitely changed my life. My body is trimmer and I am fitter than I have been in years. Dance has taken 10 years off my age, and my health has improved tremendously. Dance has also boosted my confidence, enabling me to make lots of new friends because it makes me feel good about myself. When I'm dancing I forget all my problems – it's as if I'm transported to another planet – problem free! ”

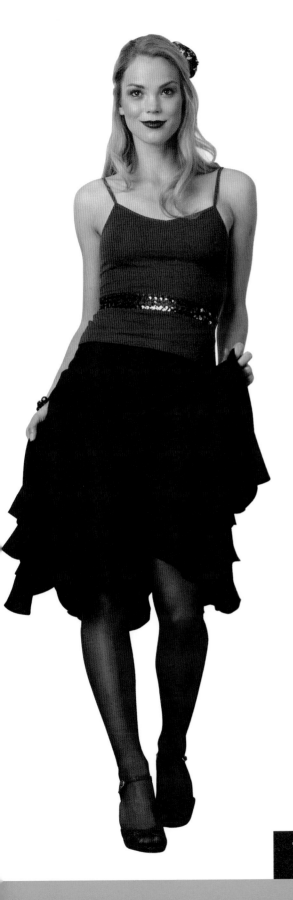
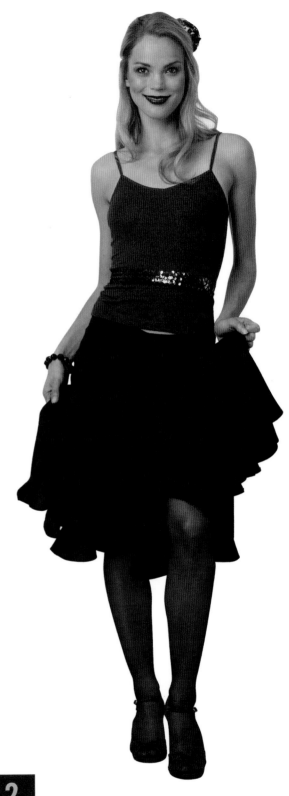

1 2

The killer move: side-front step to right and Cha Cha

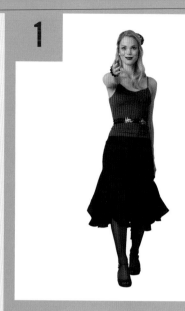

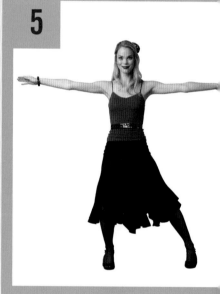

You might not have tried it before, but you've surely heard of the Cha Cha. Originally known as the Cha Cha Cha (the extra 'Cha' makes all the difference!), the move is an offshoot of the Mambo. In the slow Mambo tempo, there was a distinct sound in the music that people began dancing to, calling the step the 'Triple' Mambo. Eventually it evolved into a separate dance, known today as the Cha Cha. In this routine the Cha Cha provides the perfect opportunity to increase drama and bring attention back to the feet. So don't hold back – dance the Cha Cha with intent. Fans and flamenco costumes optional!

1–2 Step forwards on your right foot and bring your right arm forwards (**1**). Bring your left foot forwards so your feet are together. Bring your left arm forwards in line with your right arm (**2 counts**).

3–4 Step your right foot to the side (**3**), then cross your left foot behind your right foot. Open your arms out by your side – keep them there for two counts as you walk to the right (**4 AND**).

5–6 Step your left foot out to the side (**5**) and then bring it in so it is next to your right foot (**6**). When your feet are next to each other, assume the Cha Cha position and bring your hands on to your hips **(this takes two counts)**. Hold them there for the rest of the move **(a further two counts)**.

7–8 Lift the heel of your right foot up, bend your right knee and transfer the weight on to the ball of your foot. Repeat this move on your left foot, then your right foot again. In total, these three steps should take two counts of the music – they are quick (**7, 8**).

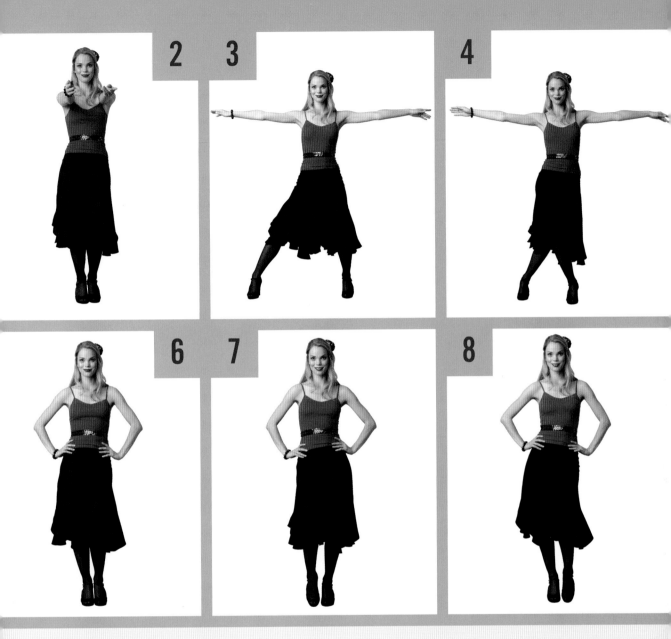

Latin is great for:

- Toning your legs – lots of the steps involve exaggerated walking so you'll soon have super-sexy pins.
- Trimming your waist and toning the abs – all the hip movements will lead you to regularly stretch your tummy muscles out, leaving you with a flatter tummy than before.
- Boosting confidence – when danced with a partner, Latin requires communication. Smile as you progress through the routine and you'll see what a difference this makes.

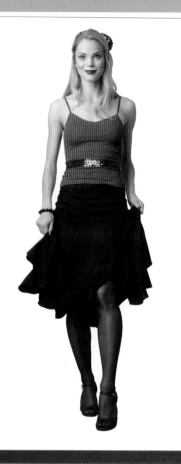

1   2

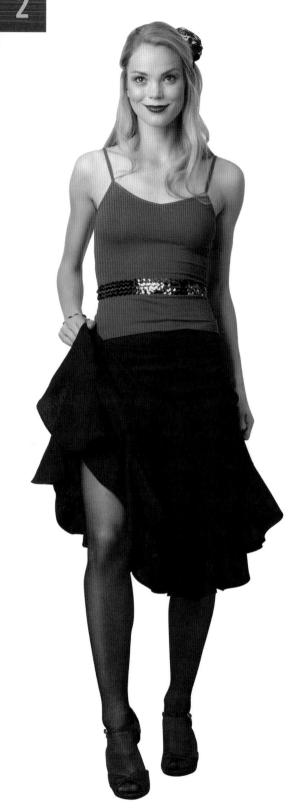

Salsa step to the left

1 Stand with your feet hip-width apart. Step your left foot forwards. Transfer the weight on to the ball of your left foot – the right heel will come off the floor. If you're wearing a skirt, you can take hold of it and swish it around as you're moving **(1)**.

2 Then step on to your right foot and take your left foot back – keep moving it past its original position and place it on the floor approximately 0.5m further back than it was at the start **(2)**.

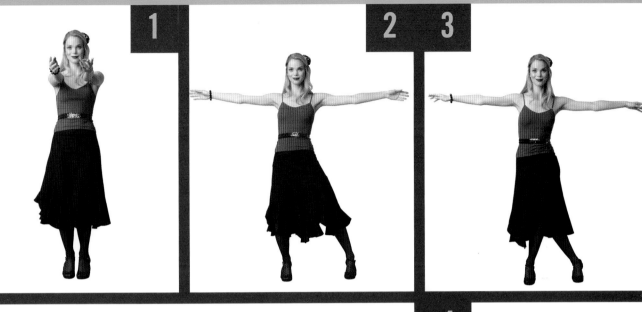

Side-front step to left and Cha Cha

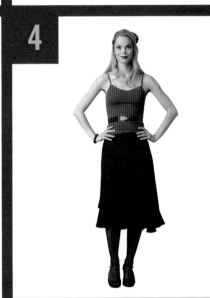

1 Step forwards on your left foot **(1)**. Bring your right foot forwards so that your feet are together. As you step on your left foot, bring your left arm forwards. Then bring your right arm forwards in time with your right foot **(2 counts)**.

2–3 Step the left foot to the side **(3)**, cross your right foot behind your left **(4)**, then step your left foot out to the side **(5)** and bring your right foot in **(6)**. Open your arms out by your sides – keep them there for two counts as you walk to the left. These four steps should take four counts of the music.

4 When your feet are next to each other facing the front, place both hands on your hips. Repeat the Cha Cha move exactly as on page 89 **(7, 8)**. As you assume the Cha Cha position, bring your hands on to your hips **(this takes 2 counts)**. Hold them there for the rest of the move **(2 more counts)**.

Turns to right and left

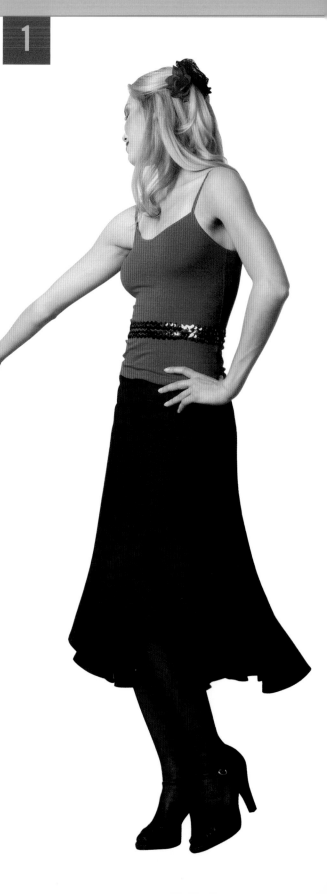

1–3 Your aim is to make a small circle with your feet, and turn your body through 360 degrees. To do this, take four mini steps with your right foot, and bring your left foot in to meet it. Each step should turn you approximately a quarter of the way around the circle, until you come back to the front again. Place your left hand on your left hip. Extend your right arm so it's pointing out and down towards the floor at a diagonal of 45 degrees. Keep your hand stretched out, nice and low, as you turn all the way round to the right **(4 counts)**.

4–5 Repeat this movement in the other direction, so you are taking four mini steps to the left, in order to turn your body all the way round in an anticlockwise direction. Place your right arm on your right hip, and extend your left arm so it's pointing up towards the ceiling at a diagonal of 45 degrees. Keep your arm extended as you turn all the way to the left **(4 counts)**.

Repeat both turns again, for another eight counts of the music.

❝ Salsa dance is my therapy. It releases my stress, tones my body and brings a huge smile to my face. I can't get enough of it! ❞

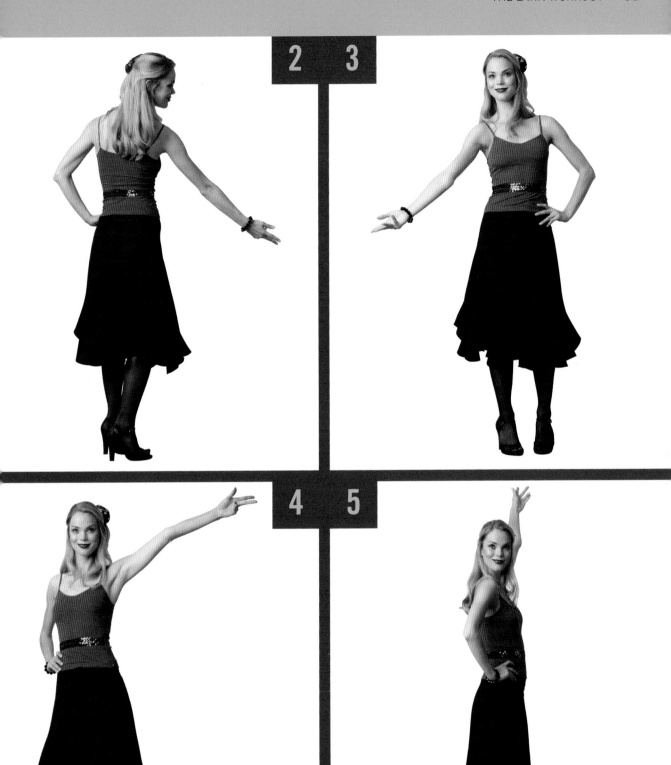

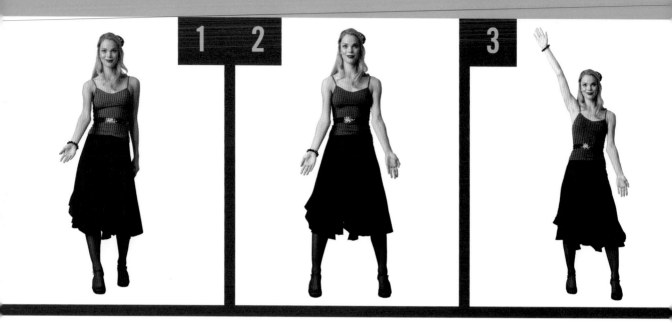

Front shimmy

1–2 Step forwards on your right foot so you are facing the front **(1)**. Then step forwards on your left foot **(2)**. As you step forwards on your right foot, bring your right arm forwards in front of you **(1)**. Then bring your left arm forwards, in time with your left foot **(2)**. Keep your head facing the front the whole time.

3–4 Step back on your right foot, then back on your left foot. As you step back on your right foot, raise your right arm into the air **(3)**. Raise your left arm as you step back on your left foot **(4)**.

5–6 Alternate your weight between left and right feet as you 'shimmy' your shoulders down. This should take four counts of the music.

7–9 Shake your shoulders rapidly in a shimmy. As you shimmy, slowly lower your arms so they end up back down by your sides. This takes four counts of the music. Enjoy yourself and let your skirt swirl around at your knees. Don't forget to smile.

Repeat this entire move again, for another eight counts of the music.

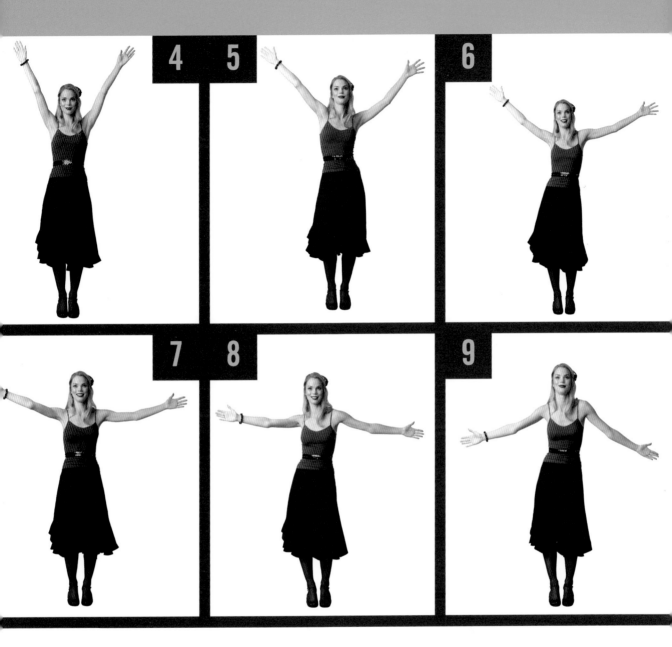

Pro tip

To shimmy like a star, keep the lower body still and suck in the tummy. Liberate the shoulders and let them float around. It will feel odd at first, but after a few attempts you'll get the drift. It's worth persevering because it looks fabulous!

Tango walk and leg flick

1 Start with your legs together and your arms slightly out at your sides, then place your hands on your hips **(1)**.

2 Lift your right leg up and flick your heel back behind you **(2)**. As you flick your right heel up, raise your left arm and point it to the ceiling **(3, 4)**. Step forwards on to your right leg. Keep your knee bent, as if making a mini lunge. Hold this pose for an extra count.

3 Make four more steps to the right side of the room, leading with your left leg. Lower your left arm as you walk across the room, and point it out in front of you. Keep your right arm bent, with your hand on your hip, at all times **(5, 6, 7, 8)**.

Pro tip

If you're finding the footwork confusing, let your arms lead you. In this routine, arms and legs work together – not in opposition – so if you can remember to stretch your right arm in front of you, your legs are sure to follow. Give it a go, and if you don't get it right first time, try again.

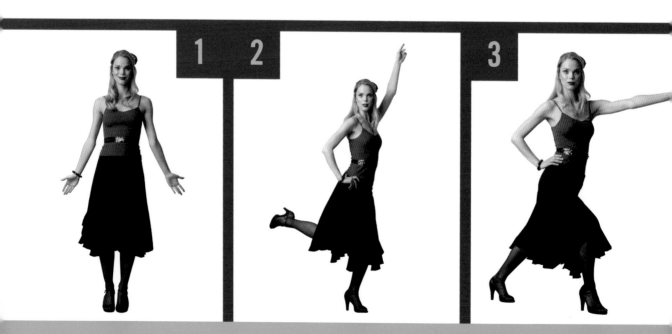

1   2   3

Walk to left

1 Start with your hands on your hips. Step to the left on your left leg **(1)**. Flick your left heel up behind you. As you flick your left heel up, raise your right arm and point it to the ceiling **(2)**.

2 Step forwards on to your left leg. Keep your knee bent, as if making a mini lunge. Hold this pose for an extra count **(3, 4)**. Then make four more steps to the right side of the room, leading with your left leg **(5 ,6 ,7 ,8)**. Lower your right arm as you walk across the room, and point it out in front of you. Keep your left arm bent, hand on hip, at all times.

When you reach the end of your walk, take four extra steps to turn you around and bring you back to face the front. Place your hands on your hips and start the routine again from the top. Keep dancing until the end of the track and let yourself go. You'll enjoy it more the second time around!

Pro tip

If you've got a partner who fancies trying this routine, ask him to stand in front of you and hold you in what's called an 'embrace'. He will need to reverse all the movements – he will be travelling to his right when you're moving to the left – but it's not too tricky to get this right. And if you pull it off, you'll feel amazing. So give it a go. If cricketer-turned-*Strictly Come Dancing* winner Darren Gough can master ballroom dancing, your man can too.

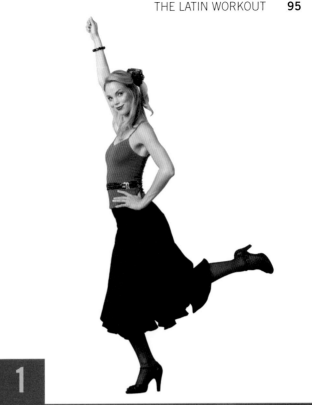

1

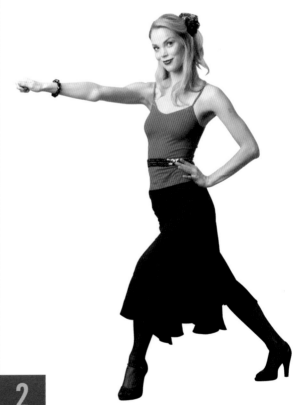

2

Choosing your music and workout level

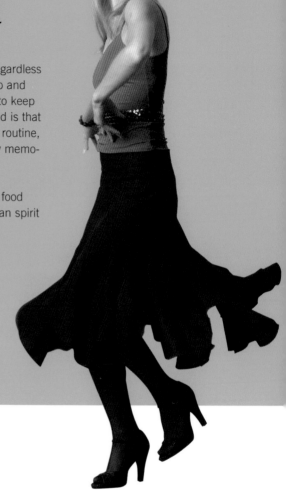

The steps in this routine should be danced the same way, regardless of your fitness level. However, if you want to spice things up and really sweat, choose a song with a quicker tempo and aim to keep pace with the music as you dance. The key thing to bear in mind is that Latin dance is all about communication. When you perform this routine, think back to your best summer holiday ever and let your happy memories guide you.

Dance clubs in South America are fuelled by hot weather, spicy food and the occasional tequila shot, so channel some South American spirit into your dance and you'll have a great time.

Latin playlists

**GETTING FIT
(level 1)**

1. Bebel Gilberto
   'August Day Song'
2. Salsa Roja
   'Girl From Ipanema'
3. Rolando Sanchez
   'Nena'

**FIGHTING FIT
(level 2)**

1. Tribalistas
   'Passe en Casa'
2. Jennifer Lopez
   'Carino'
3. Salsa Festival
   'La Belleza'

**SUPER-FIT
(level 3)**

1. Caetano Veloso
   'Onde o Rio e mas Baian'
2. Lady Salsa
   'Somos Cubanos'
3. Gloria Estefan
   'Rhythm is Gonna Get You'

Case study

Kim Schwartz, 31, began learning Tango at the age of 26, while training to be a lawyer in London. She loved the dance so much that in 2003, she moved to Argentina to throw herself into the Latin dance scene. She now lives in Buenos Aires, where she works part-time as tour manager for the internationally acclaimed dance company, Tango Por Dos.

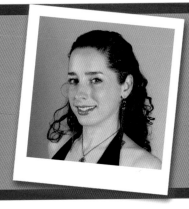

'I was 26 and when I tried tango for the first time. Back then, my life was really busy and juggling the demands of my job and a hectic social life was a struggle. I worked out at the gym three times a week, but I never saw the results I wanted. I was demotivated about exercise and constantly on diets. But the night that I went with my sister to a tango class, everything changed.

'Although I hardly knew what I was doing, I managed to follow the teachers' instructions and I fell in love with tango straight away. The meditative nature of the class was amazing. Instead of pushing papers around my desk, I was using my mind and body to tell a story. My stress literally melted away and the whole experience was very special. From then on, tango became a major part of my life. I took private lessons and went dancing six times per week. Tango quickly became a passion for me and I was determined not to let a corporate job get in the way of something I loved.

'By 2003, I was so into my tango that I decided to take a break from law and move to Argentina.

There's a thriving social scene in the Milongas – or dance clubs – in Buenos Aires, and I wanted to experience the atmosphere first hand. Living in a different country was tough at first, but I quickly got

'Dance is my miracle cure. It's completely changed my shape and got rid of the need to diet!'

used to it. Best of all, my new lifestyle allowed me to dance social tango several times per week, which has led to a complete overhaul in the way I feel about my life and my body.

'Tango has boosted my body confidence 100 per cent. I enjoy it so much it doesn't feel like I'm exercising, and yet It's my miracle cure. It's taken away my need to diet and it's helped me to lose over a stone in weight. I never thought I'd be so slim, but my body has toned up beyond belief. I was

never happy with my thighs but now I don't have insecurities about my lower body. I've also stopped comparing myself negatively to other people. I used to feel guilty for not loving yoga enough to do it four times a week, but looking back I realise I wasn't being lazy, I just hadn't found the right exercise for me.

'If you've never tried Latin dance before, you must give the routine in this book a go. Don't worry if you haven't exercised in ages. Latin dancing isn't going to zap your energy. At the end of your workout you'll feel relaxed, clearheaded and happy. It will be an hour well spent. Latin dance has opened up a whole new world to me. Give it a go and see what it can do for you!'

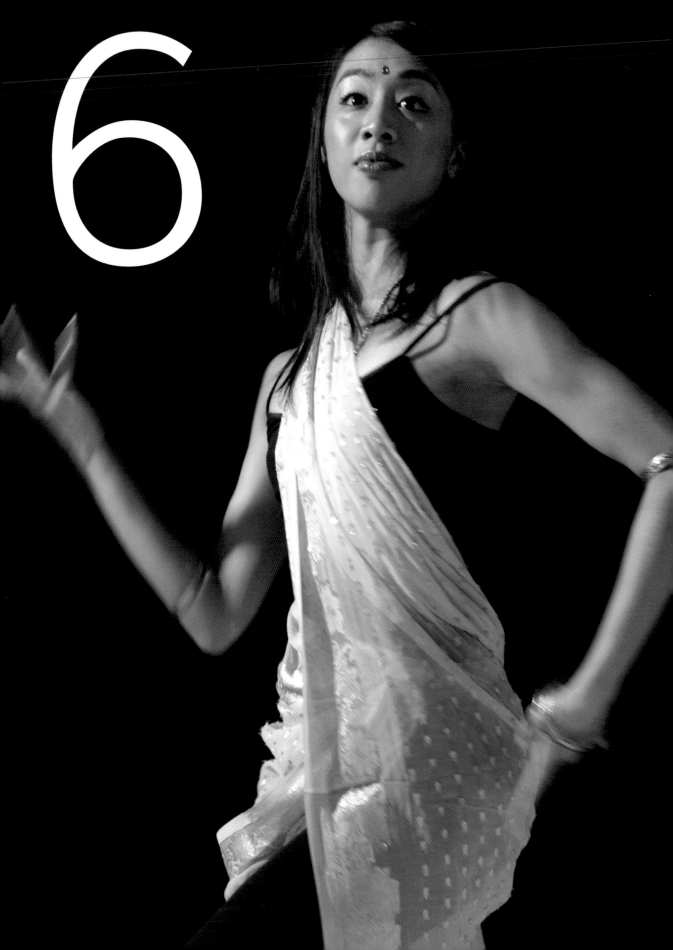

6

The Bollywood Workout

Bollywood dance is brilliant fun and very easy to pick up, but it does involve moves with names that you're unlikely to have heard of before – such as Jump Jump Heel and Double Leg Pushy Pushy. Don't be fooled by these contemporary labels, though. Modern Bollywood dance owes a lot to ancient forms of Indian classical dance, versions of which have been around since 400 BC.

At its core, Bollywood dance is a celebration of life. Indian women used to perform these moves as they harvested crops in the fields. By dancing, they were showing gratitude for a good harvest. Today, Bollywood dance has come a long way from the fields of India. The Hindi film industry is the biggest in the world – there are more Bollywood films produced every year in India than anywhere else, including Hollywood. Its actors are international superstars, much feted across the globe for their good looks, smooth skin and amazing dance skills.

The workout on the following pages is devised by David Olton, a man who performed in the West End in Andrew Lloyd Webber's Bollywood musical, *Bombay Dreams*. He's put a selection of moves together which will make you sweat and get you fit. So pick a tune from the custom-built Bollywood playlist and get dancing…

> **' Bollywood dance is a celebration of life. It's a brilliant way of getting fit and it's easy to pick up and great fun. '**

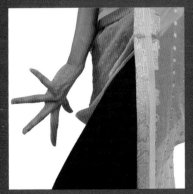
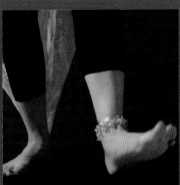
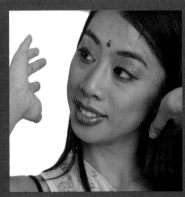

Indian classical hands

This classical hand position crops up several times during this routine, so get the hang of it before you begin. It will make things easier.

Stand with your legs together and stretch your arms out wide. Roll your hands over so that your palms are facing the ceiling. Splay your fingers, and lift your little finger so that it is higher than all your other fingers. Your thumb should be pointing downwards.

In Indian classical dance, this move signifies the question 'Why?'. It is incorporated into many of the moves in this routine, so master it early on and you'll be off to a good start!

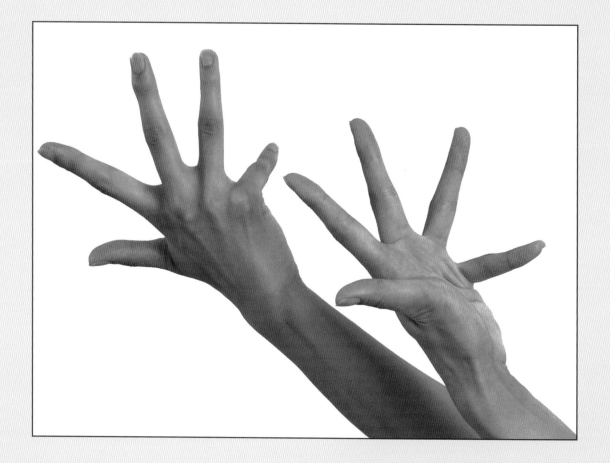

Indian bop step

1 Stand with your left leg bent and lifted off the floor. Face the left-hand diagonal of the room. Holding your hands away from you, roll your shoulders backwards and forwards, as if in time to the beat of a drum.

2 Stretch both arms out to the left, so they are pointing in the same direction as your legs. Twist your palms, as explained in the Indian classical hands (left), although in this move your hands will move in opposite directions (your right hand will move clockwise, your left hand anticlockwise). Bend your elbows slightly and point your fingers. Practise straightening and bending your arms in quick succession. When your elbows are bent, your hands are nearer to your face than when the arms are straight.

❛ There's something magic about Bollywood dancing, it's that rush of adrenaline I love. It makes me feel so alive! ❜

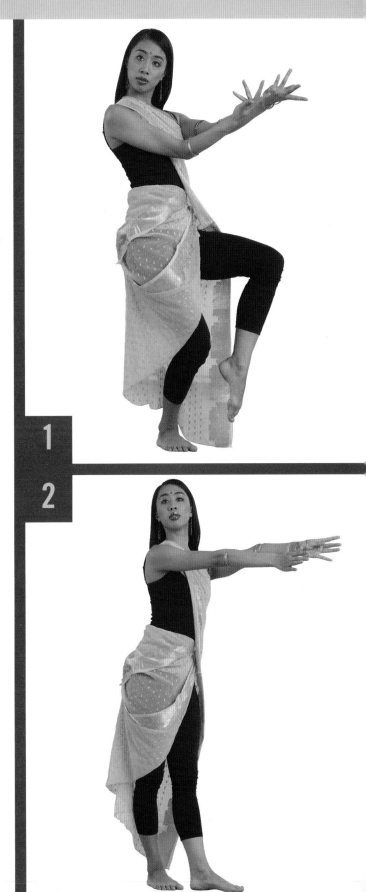

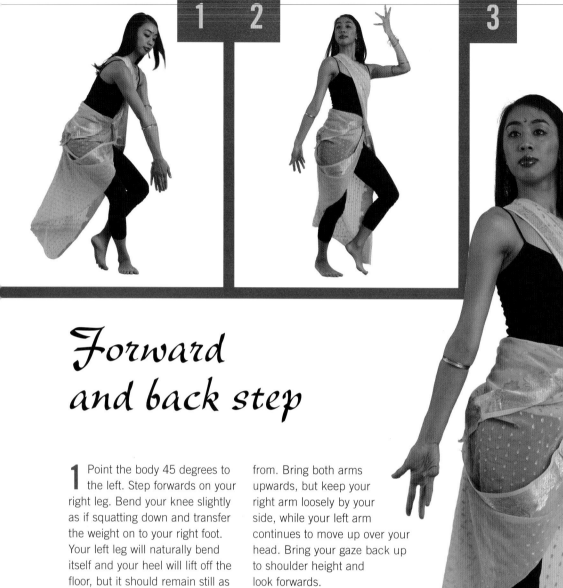

Forward and back step

1 Point the body 45 degrees to the left. Step forwards on your right leg. Bend your knee slightly as if squatting down and transfer the weight on to your right foot. Your left leg will naturally bend itself and your heel will lift off the floor, but it should remain still as much as possible. Bend forwards from your hips, stretch your arms out and clap your hands together in front of your knees. Allow your eyes to follow your body. Move your head to your left and look to the floor.

2 Step on to your right leg and lift your left leg up. This is a mini step, designed to get you ready to put your left leg back on the floor, exactly where it came

from. Bring both arms upwards, but keep your right arm loosely by your side, while your left arm continues to move up over your head. Bring your gaze back up to shoulder height and look forwards.

3 Step your right foot back behind your left leg and straighten your right leg. When your left hand reaches your left ear, stop and rest it just behind your head. When your left hand is in position, flick your right hand 45 degrees anticlock-wise, so that your little finger is at the front and your palm is facing upwards (see Indian Classical Hands on page 100).

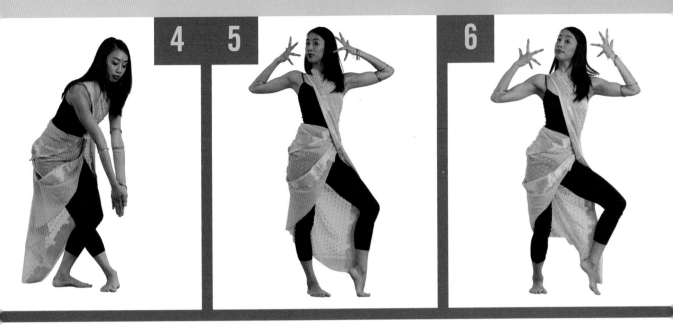

4 Bend forwards from your hips, stretch your arms out and clap your hands together in front of your knees. Lower your gaze to your hands.

5 Move both arms up to head level and circle your right arm around the back of your head. Place your right hand behind your right ear and your left hand behind your left ear.

6 When your hands are in the right place, rotate your wrists 45 degrees anticlockwise and look forwards: it's as though you're flicking your wrists and making direct eye contact with the front. At this point your body should be facing forwards.

Pro tip

The moves above should work together as a continuous motion. Practise it – we're going to be dancing it four times!

The legs work in exactly the same way as outlined in moves 1–3. The difference with moves 4–6 is that both hands end up on either side of the head, and the face is looking forwards.

Killer move: jump jump heel

1 Do two mini jumps to the left. After the second jump, straighten your right leg and flex your foot. Stretch both arms out to the right. Flex your hands so your palms are facing the wall, away from your face.

2 Slowly move your right leg back so that your feet are together. Keeping your arms straight, move them all the way across your body until they are pointing to the left-hand side.

3 Turn your left hand 45 degrees to the left, and your right hand 45 degrees to the right. Bend your elbows slightly. This is called a 'pully', and it completes the move by giving it some traditional finesse.

To add some variety to the move, you can change the movement of your arms (step 4 or 5).

4 Alternative move 1. With palms facing away from you, bring your arms over your head instead of across your chest. Then flick your wrists as before.

5 Alternative move 2. Move your arms from left to right by moving them underneath your chest, and bring them together on your right-hand side of your face. Look forwards and clap twice in celebration of your fabulous coordination!

6 Repeat your move on the left-hand side. Straighten your left leg and flex your foot. Bring your arms together on the left-hand side of your face and clap.

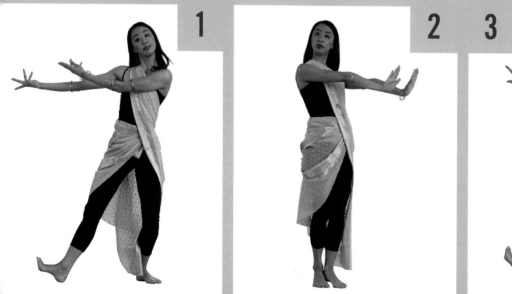

1

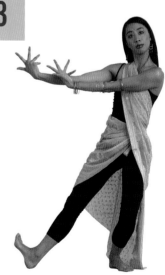

2 3

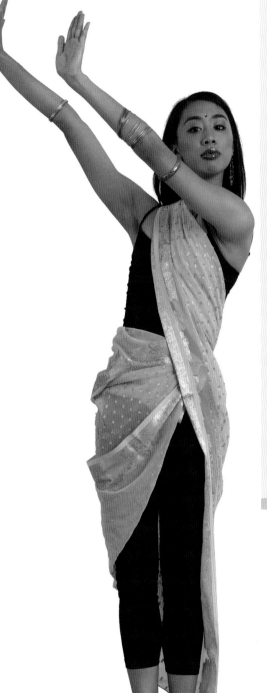

4

Pro tip

Clapping twice might feel odd because you're only kicking your foot out once. Don't worry about this imbalance – it's how all top Bollywood dancers execute the move. My top tip for getting it right? Practise, practise and practise some more! Once you've cracked it, you'll feel brilliant. The move is great for raising the heart rate and increasing coordination. It comes up several times in this routine so it's a good idea to master it early on.

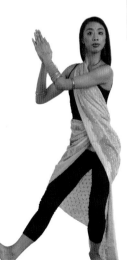

5

6

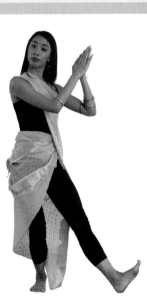

Double leg pushy pushy

1 Start with both legs straight and your feet together.

2–3 Lift your right leg off the floor and kick forwards from below your knee. Repeat this kick twice without stopping. Your arms basically follow the direction of your legs. Here's what to do:

Keep your right arm by your side, but splay your fingers and move your arm out 30 degrees, so it's hanging at a slight angle. Bend your left arm and place your hand behind the left side of your head. Both arms move forwards when your leg is kicked forwards, and move back when your leg is taken backwards.

4 This time, lift your left leg off the floor and kick forwards from below your knee. Repeat this move twice without stopping. With your left arm out at 30 degrees, bend your right arm and place your hand behind the right side of your head.

5 As you kick your left leg forwards, move your left arm forwards and splay your fingers. Move your right elbow forwards, but keep your right hand near your head.

Repeat the move eight times, alternating between left and right.

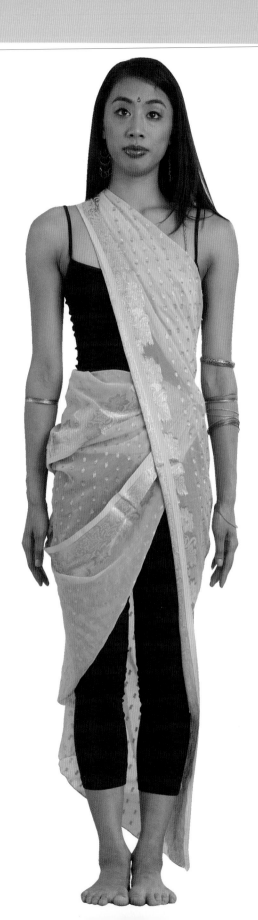

1

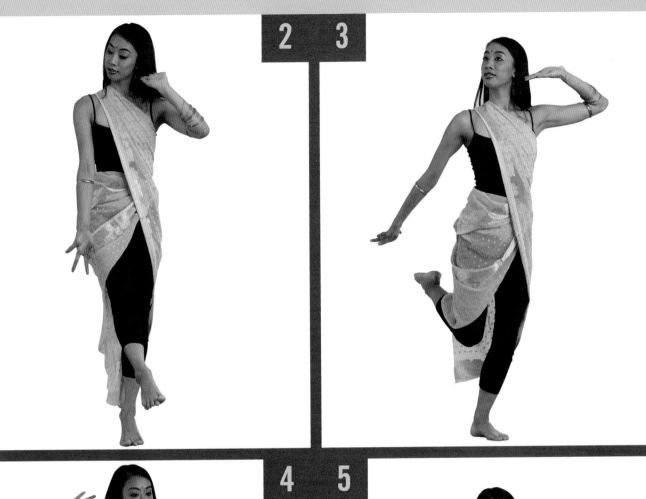

2   **3**

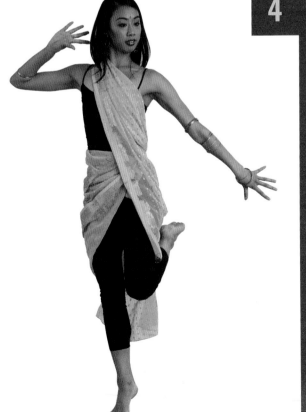

4   **5**

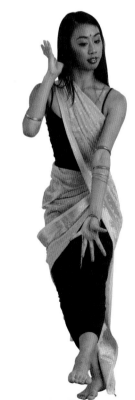

Twists

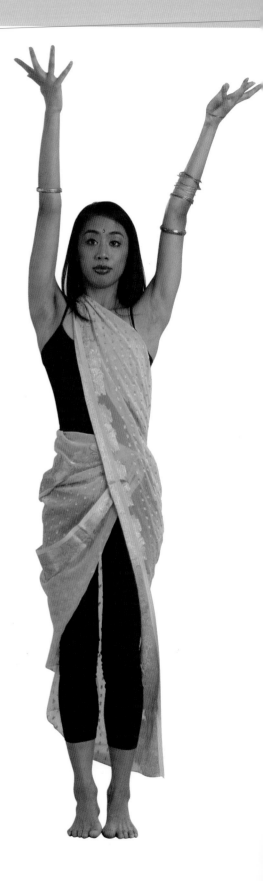

1 Face the front with your feet together. Place your arms in the air above your head.

2 Jump on the spot and allow your heels to turn out to the left – your bottom should follow. As you twist your heels out to the left, bring your arms down and move them out to the left. Repeat this move eight times on the spot.

3 By the end of all eight twists, your arms should be back by your hips.

Bollywood is great for:

- Burning fat from your hips – jumping on the spot will make you sweat.
- Increasing coordination – it's not easy at first, but after a couple of attempts you'll be moving arms and legs in sync.
- Toning your arms – keeping the arms in the air for such a long time in this routine is a guaranteed tricep toner!

2   3

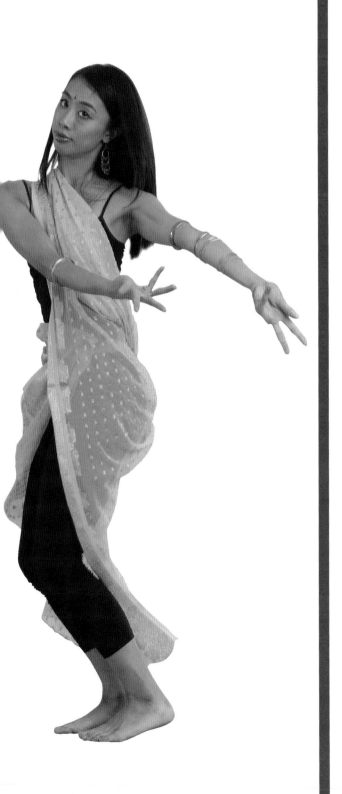
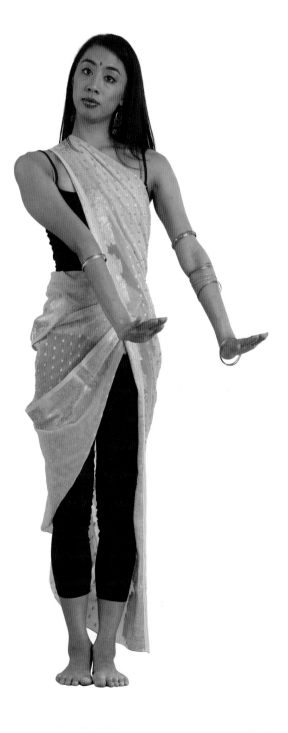

Shunting

1 **Basic shunt:** Face the front of the room. Twist your arms, place your hands on either side of your head and keep your feet together. Jump forwards and backwards in quick succession. Your body's focus is totally forwards.

Repeat eight times.

2 **Right shunt:** You're going to jump back and forwards as before, except that this time, you are facing the left side of the room and as you jump back, flick your right calf up behind you. Your left arm should be behind your head; your right arm down by your side. As you kick your right leg back, pull your right arm back too.

3 When you jump forwards, bring your right arm forwards, and your left elbow forwards (as before). Imagine that your hand is pushing your leg, and suddenly a tricky move is dead easy.

Repeat four times

4 **Left shunt:** Jump back and forwards as before, except that this time you are facing right and as you jump back, flick your left calf up behind you. Your right arm should be behind your head; your left arm down by your side.

5 As you kick your left leg back, pull your left arm back too. And when you jump forwards, bring your right arm forwards, and your left elbow forwards (as before).

Repeat four times.

6 After shunting to the left, return to the centre and repeat the basic shunt as in step 1.

Repeat eight times.

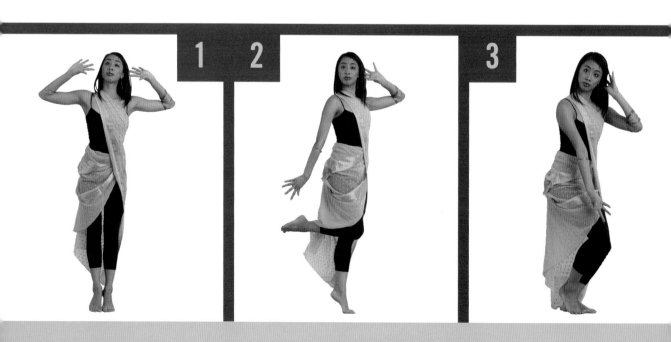

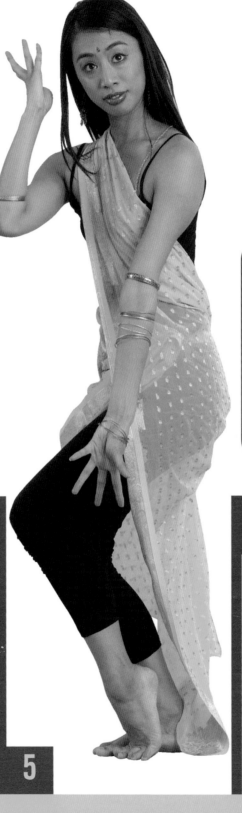

Pro tip

This is a super-simple move that's great for raising the heart rate. To increase the intensity of your workout, add sixteen shunts to your routine instead of the standard eight. You'll soon feel the extra burn.

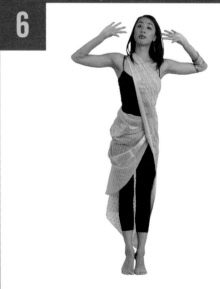

4

5

6

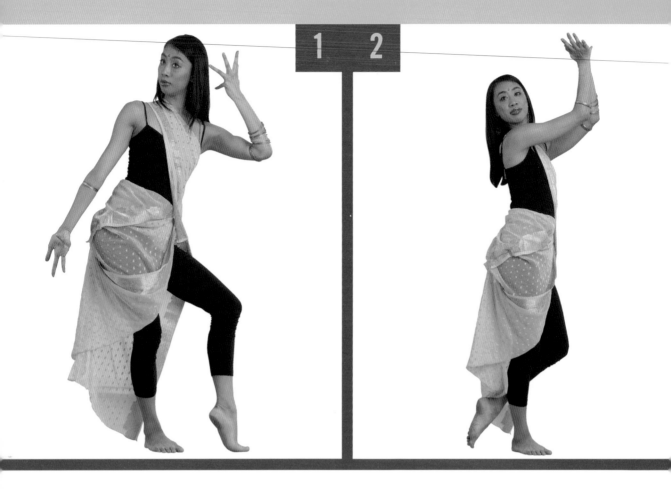

The bangle

1 Step your right foot in front of your left foot, so you are facing the left diagonal of the room. Bend your knee and transfer your weight on to your right leg. Keep your right arm down by your right hip and bend your left arm to 45 degrees with your hand by your ear.

2 As you step forwards on your right foot, bang your wrists together above your head. Bring your right leg back to where it came from. As you step back on your right foot and face your front, place your right hand on your right hip and flick your wrist outwards 45 degrees anticlockwise.

3 Step your left foot in front of your right foot, so you are facing your right diagonal of the room. As you step forwards on your left foot, bang your wrists together above your head.

4 Bend your knee and transfer your weight on to your left leg. Bring your left leg back to where it came from. As you step back on your left foot and face the front, place your left hand near your left hip, and turn your wrist outwards 45 degrees anticlockwise. Repeat this move four times to the right, four times to the left, then twice right and twice left.

3   **4**

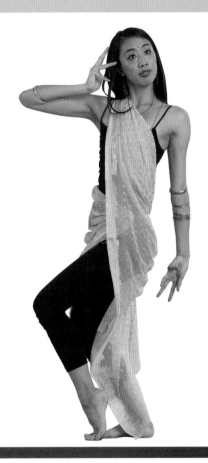

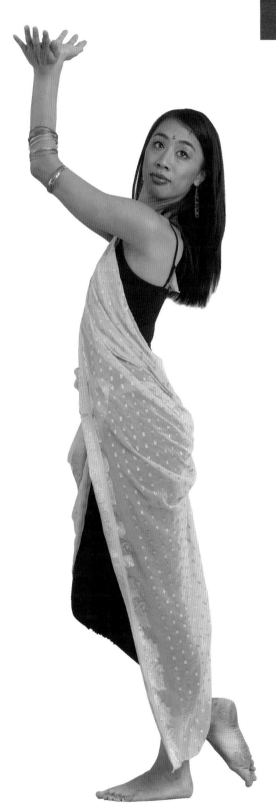

Pro tip

This move gets its name because it involves the wrist and ankle – two places where Indian women traditionally wear bangles and jewels. Bear this detail in mind and it will help you remember what to do with your hands and feet!

Leg drops

1 Face the front with your feet together. Start with the arms down by your side.

2 With your right leg as straight as you can comfortably keep it, gently lean back and in time with the music, lift your left leg off the floor (don't think of this move as a 'leg lift' – think of it more as a 'drop backwards' where your knee takes care of itself). Stretch your arms out wide and splay your fingers.

Every time you lift your leg off the floor, slowly lift your arms higher and higher into the air. Twist the hands as you go (remember Indian Classical Hands on page 100).

Pro tip

As this is an on-the-spot move, use the Leg Drop as an opportunity to take some deep breaths. By now your heartrate will be pretty high and you'll have worked up a good sweat. Breathe deeply at this point – this will stop you feeling dizzy or tired.

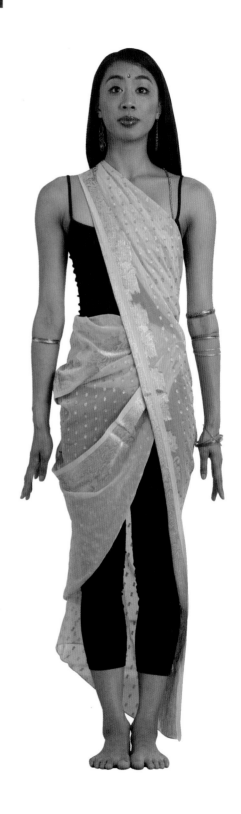

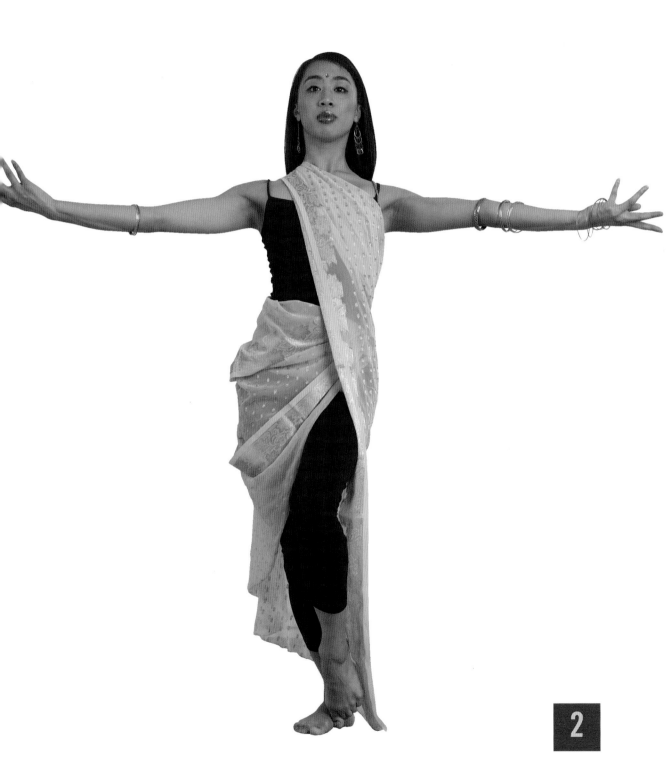

2

Bollywood twist

1 Shake your feet from left to right by jumping on the spot. Slowly bring your arms up over your head.

2 Gradually turn your body towards the left-hand side of the room, but keep your eyes looking to the front. As you are turning, slowly lower your arms and keep them stretched out with your left arm pointing towards the front. Shake your fingers a few times.

3 Face the front. Bend your left knee so that your heel lifts off the floor; keep your right leg as straight as you comfortably can. Bend your elbows and splay your fingers close to your head.

4 Move your left leg back to the centre. Bring both arms together above your head and let your wrists touch gently together. Splay your fingers, stand tall and smile. You've just completed your first Bollywood dance routine!

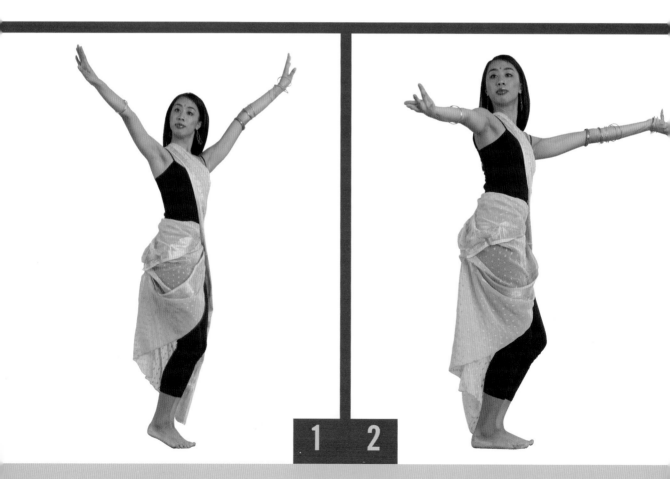

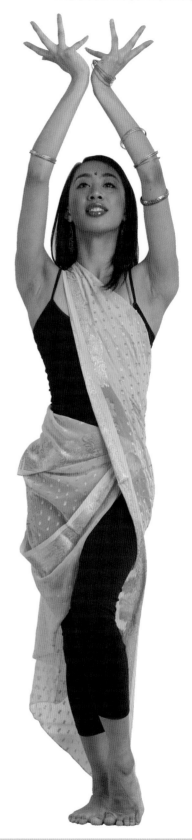

"If I didn't dance Bhangra I would not be as fit as I am, nor as energetic. It amazes people how fit dancing has actually made me – for this reason alone, I'll never stop dancing."

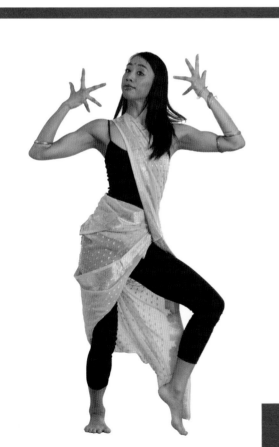

3 4

Choosing your music and workout level

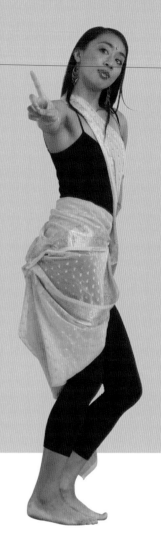

There are no two ways about it: dancing these moves to a banging Bhangra beat will make you sweat! The good news is that this routine is absolutely brilliant for increasing your cardio fitness level and toning the arms and legs. Certain moves are intended to be repeated in reps of eight, but these can be decreased or increased depending on your fitness level. Dance all the moves in a continuous movement without stopping for five minutes between moves. They're organized in a way that will increase your heartrate and then give you recovery time, so don't worry about getting out of breath.

Bollywood playlists

GETTING FIT
(level 1)

Indian Bop Step – 4 reps
Forward / Back Step – 4 reps
Jump Jump Heel – 2 reps on left, 2 reps on right
Double Leg Pushy Pushy – 4 reps on left, 4 reps on right
Twists – 4 reps on left, 4 reps on right
Shunts – 4 to the left; 4 to the front; 4 to the right
The Bangle – 2 reps to left, 2 reps to right
Leg Drops: 4 reps
Final Pose – as directed in text

FIGHTING FIT
(level 2)

Indian Bop Step – 6 reps
Forward / Back Step – 6 reps
Jump Jump Heel – 4 reps on left, 4 reps on right
Double Leg Pushy Pushy – 6 reps on left, 6 reps on right
Twists – 6 reps left; 6 reps right
Shunts – 6 to left; 6 to front; 6 to right
The Bangle – 4 to left; 4 to right
Leg Drops: 6 reps
Final Pose – as directed in text

SUPER-FIT
(level 3)

Indian Bop Step – 8 reps
Forward / Back Step – 8 reps
Jump Jump Heel – 4 on left, 4 on right
Double Leg Pushy Pushy – 8 reps left, 8 reps right
Twists – 8 reps left, 8 reps right
Shunts – 8 to left, 8 to front, 8 to right
The Bangle – 6 to left, 6 to right
Leg Drops – 8 reps
Final Pose – as directed in text

Case study

Sejal Sedani, 23, works in the healthcare industry in London. She used Bollywood dance to get her fitness and self-confidence back after student living took its toll while at university...

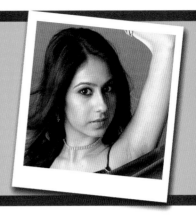

'I've always loved dance more than any other form of exercise, but when I went to university in London, I grew lazy and lost myself in student life. I'm 5ft 1in tall and I naturally have a small frame, but due to my non-existent exercise regime, I developed a thicker waist and fleshier thighs than I'd ever had before. I avoided getting on the scales because I didn't want to know what I weighed. But from trying on clothes that had become too tight and getting breathless when I ran for buses, I knew that my fitness level had gone down.

'Eventually, I realized that to get my body-confidence back, I'd need to start exercising again. I went to a Bollywood dance class at a London studio and felt better just for stepping into the room. It was like coming home!

'Within a few days of restarting dance, my confidence had increased and my general lust for life had started to flood back. I kept going, and within three months my abs were more toned, my waist had slimmed down and my pot belly had started to decrease. I've always loved tight clothes and bright colours, so to celebrate my new-look figure, I went out and bought a short top that flaunts my stomach. Wearing it for the first time was scary but it gave me a thrill, too. Nowadays I can dance all night long (and run

'Bollywood dancing is about emotions, so really give it your all.'

for a bus) without getting tired. I have a healthier, more positive outlook on life and I owe a lot of this to Bollywood dancing.

'Bollywood is an energetic form of dance and just ten minutes of dance is enough to move me into a happy state. After a class, I can never stop smiling! This is because Bollywood is a really entertaining, fun form of dance. It's also a very feminine dance form and hence is a great way for women to explore their femininity. My tip for anyone wanting to give this workout a go is to be brave and try it.

'Bollywood dancing is all about emotions, so really give it your all. Invite some friends over and make your Bollywood workout a social event. Put on some coloured clothes and lose yourself in Bhangra music. No one is too uncoordinated to dance Bollywood – it is for people of all different levels and abilities, and it will reshape your body, too.'

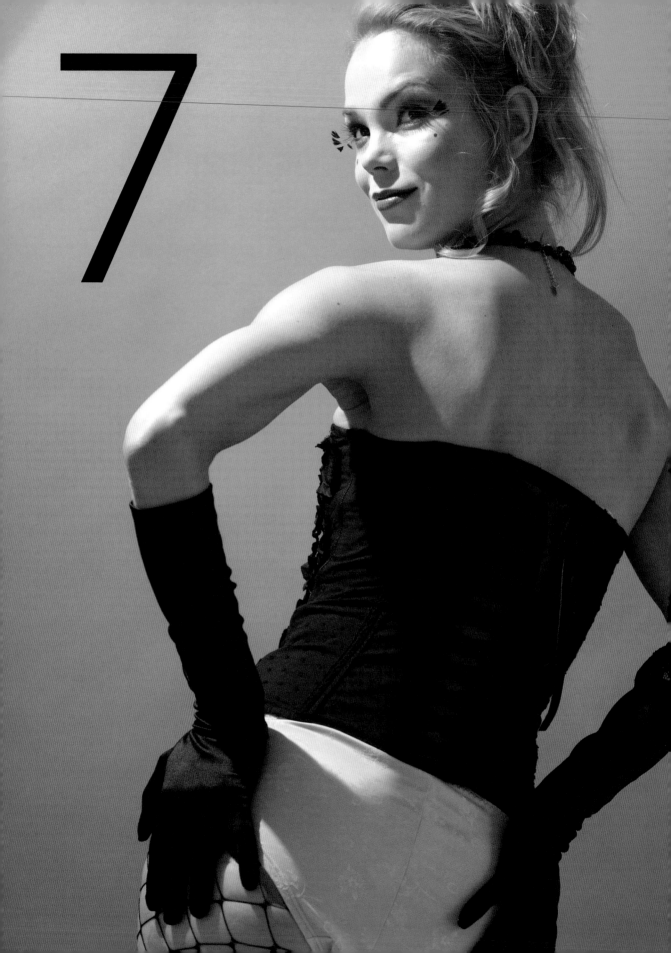

7

The Burlesque Workout

Burlesque was born in the jazz clubs and cabaret bars of 1920s America, at a time when mainstream society was terribly scared of striptease. At clubs such as Minsky's and Little Apollo in New York, showgirls would waltz on stage, swing their hips, flash their flesh and tease the assembled male audience to their heart's content. The femme fatale ruled the roost in the 1920s, with women such as Josephine Baker and Mae Dix making their mark. By the 1930s, Gypsy Rose Lee had become the queen of Burlesque.

Skip forward more than 70 years to 2007 and the world is in the grip of an international Burlesque revival. Spurred on by the satin-skinned, super-sexy Dita Von Teese – who lives her life by highly glamorous rules – Burlesque clubs are opening up all across the UK. Burlesque dance is acknowledged to be a fabulous way to increase confidence, tone the body and hone flirting skills in the process. A-listers including Gwen Stefani, Eva Longoria and Charlize Theron have all taken to the stage at Burlesque clubs in LA, as well as dancers-turned-singers, the Pussycat Dolls.

Crucially though, Burlesque is not about stripping, so banish those naked-body nerves right now! Burlesque is about glamour, glitz and old-school girly fabulousness. It's totally different to Hip Hop and Bollywood, but will leave you feeling just as exhilarated and adrenaline-fuelled. So leave your inhibitions at the door, ladies, and give it a go!

> **Burlesque dancing is a fabulous way to increase confidence, tone your body and hone your flirting skills.**

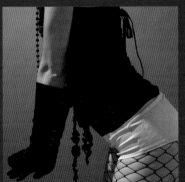
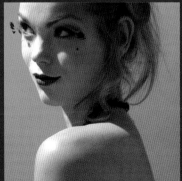
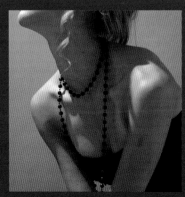

Pose and wiggle

1 Place your right arm behind your head and place your left hand on your left hip. Bend your left knee. Then move your hips from side to side, so they wiggle up and down, in time to the music. Repeat this move four times.

2–4 Stop moving and pose, looking your audience in the eye. Stretch your right arm up to the ceiling and then gradually move it down in a circular motion to rest it on your hip. This should take a minimum of five seconds, but to make the move more dramatic, you can make it take longer.

Pro tip

Dance in front of a mirror. Mirrors are useful for all types of dancing, but none more so than Burlesque. You might feel too body-conscious to watch yourself in the mirror at first, but it is best to conquer this fear as soon as possible and swap a blank wall for a room with a full-length mirror in. As soon as you catch sight of yourself looking sexy, you'll realize that you do have a Burlesque temptress lurking inside you. She might need some TLC to help her emerge, but if you experiment with facial expressions, make-up and dance moves in front of the mirror, you'll soon work out what's hot – and what's not – for you. So dust off that mirror and get dancing!

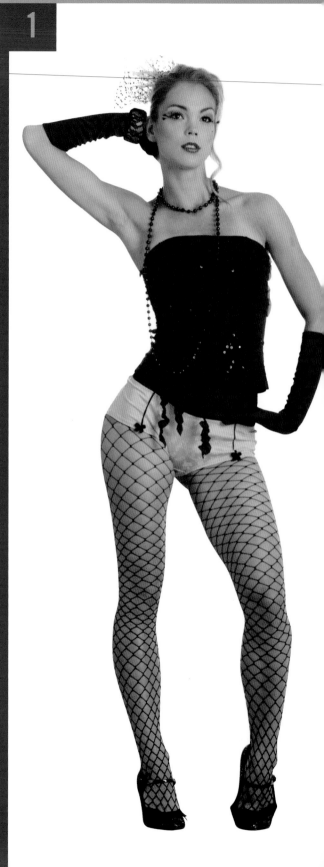

1

2 **3**

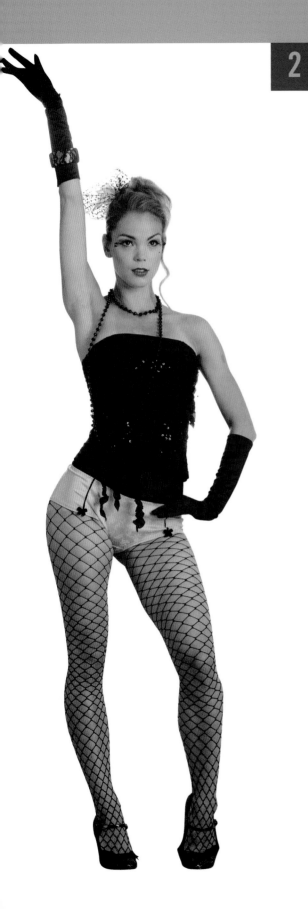

4

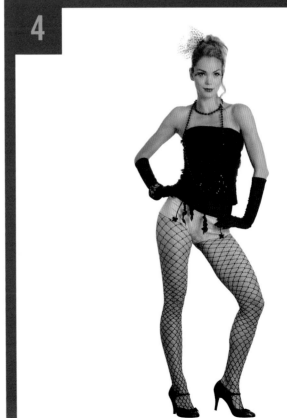

Wiggle and side bumps

1 Move your hips from side to side. Your hips should lead your body, and your legs should remain stationary, but bend at your knees. Make the movements slow and exaggerated, and repeat the move six times. Keep your hands on your hips.

2 Shake things up with a side bump. To do this, move your hips dramatically from side to side. First thrust them to the right, then the left. Once your hip is pointing outwards, stand still and look at the mirror or your audience. This is a dramatic moment in the dance, so be proud of your physique and let your body do the talking.

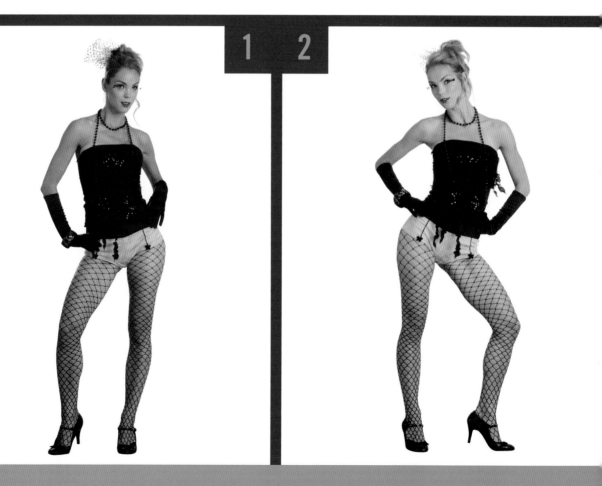

Walk and front four-step

1 Walk forwards for eight steps. Start with your right leg, and let your arms sway naturally as you move.

2–3 Starting with your right leg, draw a rectangular box with your foot. To do this, move your right foot forwards, then your left foot out to the side. Then move your right foot back, and your left foot out to the side. This is called a four-step.

Repeat this move twice.

Pro tip

To make your walk ultra-feminine, lead with your hips and tilt your pelvis backwards as you move. Look the 'audience' – or mirror – in the eye, and flirt as you walk. Imagining you are being watched will help you to pull your pelvis in and stand tall, like a showgirl. Fabulous!

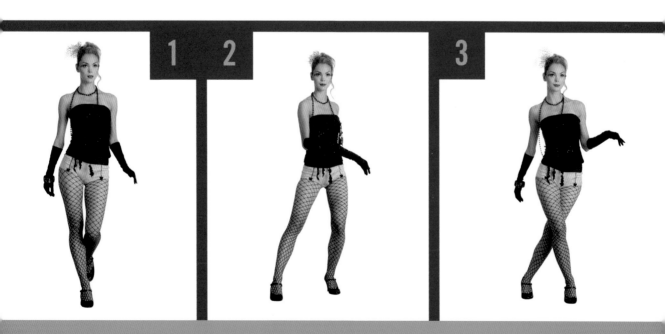

Side steps

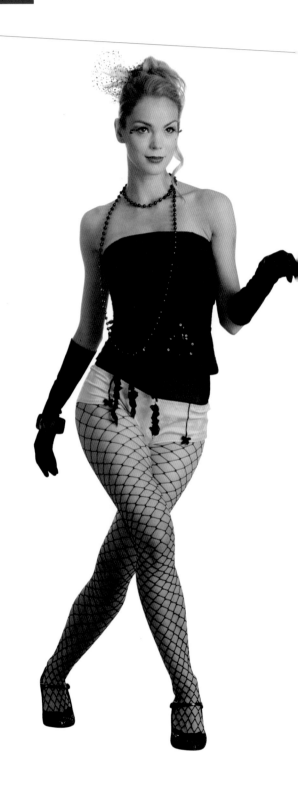

1 Leading with your right leg, walk diagonally to the left for two steps. Flick your head dramatically as you move. Let your arms float naturally.

2 Wiggle your hips four times whilst shaking your arms around seductively.

3 Repeat this move in the other direction. So start with your left leg and walk four steps, diagonally, to the right. Then wiggle your hips four times whilst shaking your arms around seductively, as before.

Burlesque is great for:

- Toning thighs – all that slow, sexy walking will tone and invigorate the tops of your legs.
- Increasing confidence – once you've danced in a corset and fishnets you'll be able to cope with all of life's little challenges. I promise!
- Loosening your hips – hidden tensions will soon disappear as your hips become more and more relaxed.

2   3

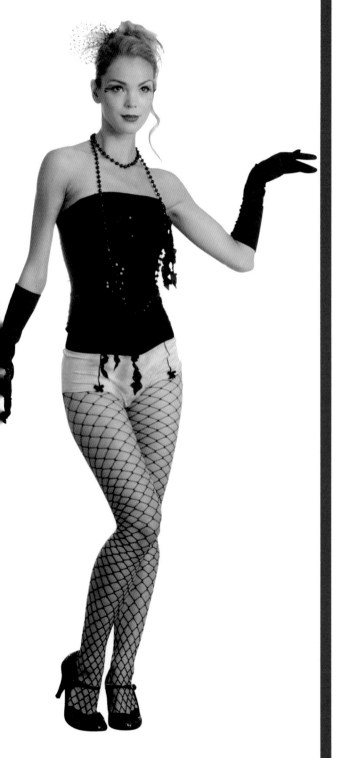
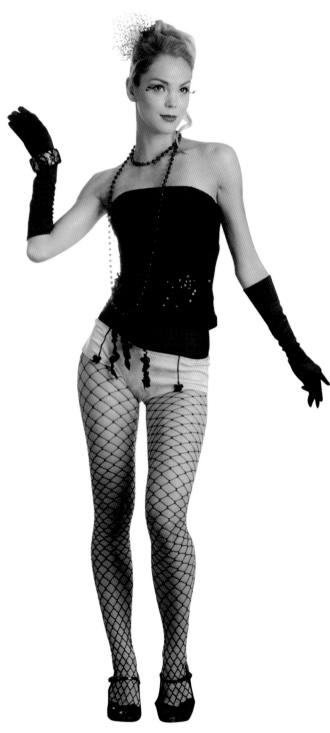

Arms up and over the body

1–4 Standing still with your legs straight, fan your arms up and in a circular motion until your hands are above your head.

5–6 Open your arms and bring your hands slowly back down, gently touching the outline of your body as they move. Keep your fingers gently splayed. Slightly tilt your body forwards, but keep your head back.

7–8 Once your hands reach your hips, straighten your head, wiggle your body twice from right to left and wink at your audience.

Pro tip

Let your eyes follow your hands in this routine. Glancing at your body as you dance will encourage you to really perform. It will also help you to fall in love with your own body – a vital attribute for all Burlesque dancers.

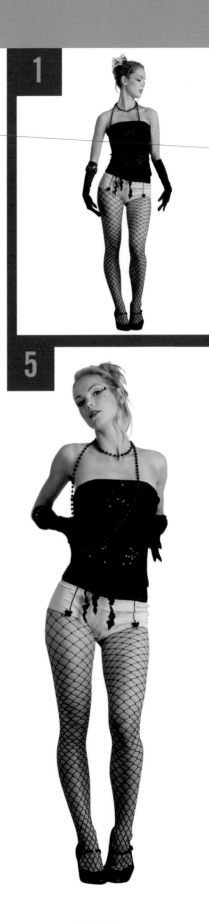

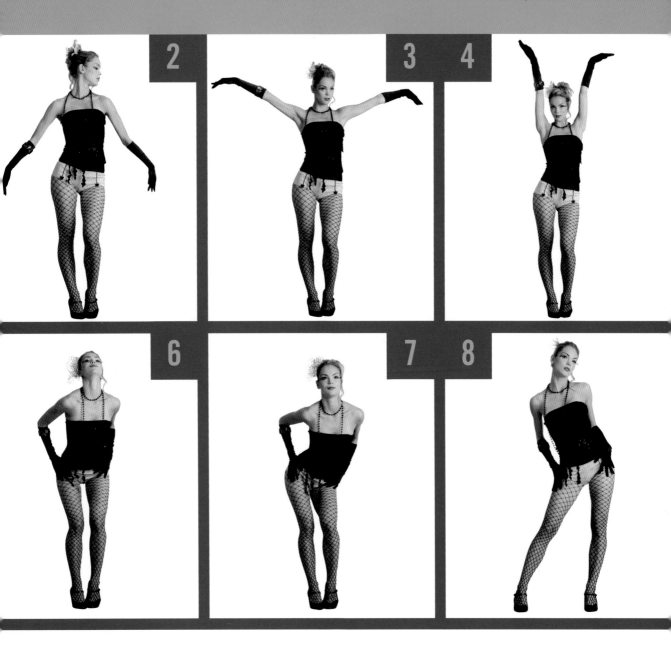

"After six weeks of Burlesque dancing, I feel sexy, liberated, and lots of people have noticed I have my "sparkle" back. Burlesque is a lot more than a bit of fun – it's a life makeover."

Killer move: grinding and front bumps

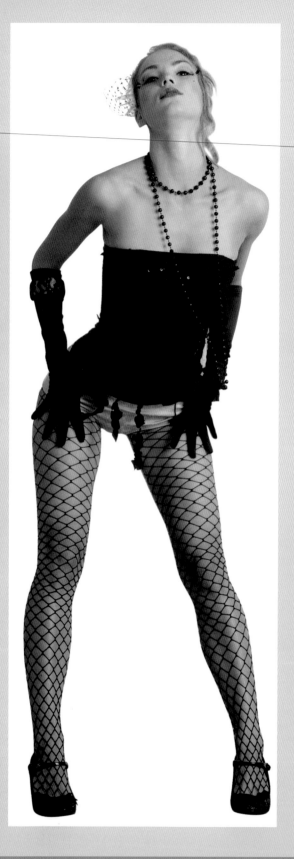

This move is an exaggerated version of your hip wiggle. It's fabulous for loosening your hips and works dramatic wonders midway through a Burlesque act. The front bumps are cheeky and fun – in many ways, they're in stark contrast to the dramatic grinds that form the first part of the move. It sounds scary but it's a great move to try. So loosen up and give it a go!

1 Tilt your pelvis forwards and rotate your hips as though drawing a circle with your bottom. Alternate between moving your stomach forwards and leaning backwards, and bending your chest forwards and sticking your bottom out. Keep your face relaxed and your hands on your hips, fingers splayed.

Repeat this move three times, and exaggerate the movements with every repetition.

Place your arms at a 45 degree angle away from your body and splay your fingers. Stand still and then suddenly move your pelvis forwards six times, as if knocking something over with your belly button.

Grind turn

1 Move your arms over your head and wiggle your fingers.

2–3 Keeping your arms up in the air, rotate your feet in small circles and turn your body around. Do this by leading with your left leg and turning in a clockwise direction.

Pro tip

Make your grind turns as dramatic and exaggerated as you dare! The bigger your hip movements, the greater the spectacle for anyone watching. But don't forget to flirt with your arms too. Fingers shouldn't flop all over the place – instead they should be nicely elongated and super-sexy.

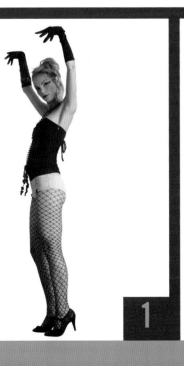

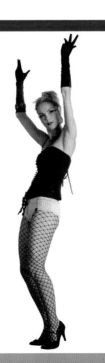

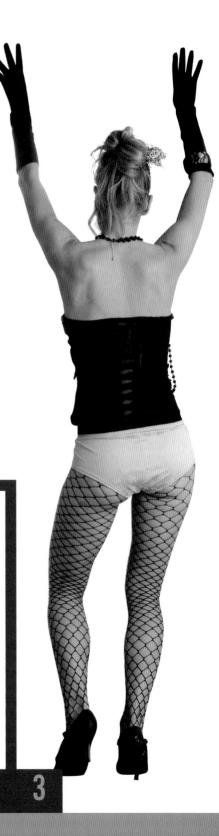

1

2 3

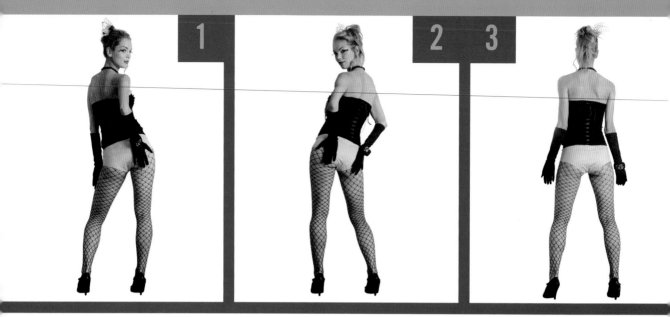

Bottom shimmy

1 Slap both hands on to your buttocks and shake your bottom very fast!

2–3 Do this by quickly lifting your heels off the floor and tapping them back down super-quick. In five seconds you should be able to tap the floor 15 times.

4–7 Start to turn back to face the front, by flicking your left foot forwards and pivoting on the right until you are front-facing again. Keep your arms above your head while you do this, flicking them as you go.

8–9 When you reach the front again, lower your arms and take four exaggerated steps to the front.

Pro tip

Don't waste time worrying about cellulite, VPL or any other bottom-related blushes. Curves are a precious commodity in Burlesque dance, and any move that gives a girl the opportunity to flaunt her fabulousness should be embraced.

So in the spirit of old-school Burlesque, shake it, baby, and leave your self-consciousness in the dressing room.

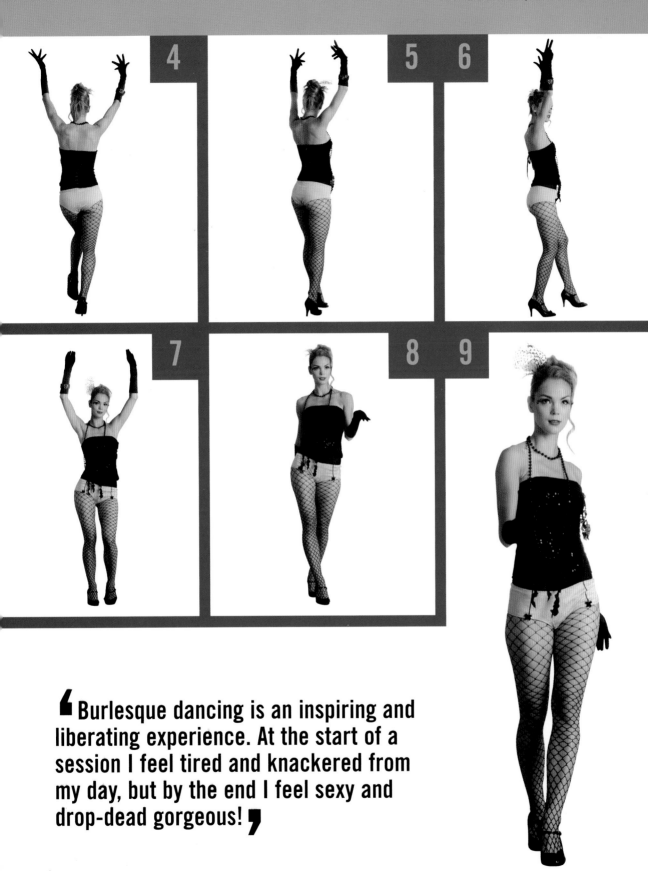

4 5 6 7 8 9

"Burlesque dancing is an inspiring and liberating experience. At the start of a session I feel tired and knackered from my day, but by the end I feel sexy and drop-dead gorgeous!"

Framing, caressing and posing

1 Face the right-hand corner of the room, bend your right leg and reach your hands down towards the floor. Don't worry about touching your toes – just reach for a point on your body that is comfortable.

2 Slowly slide your hands up the front of your body. When they reach chest height, turn to the left-hand corner of the room and repeat the move in the opposite direction, bending your left leg and reaching down over it.

3 Finish your caress with a dramatic pose. Arms can be over your head, on hips – wherever you like. But savour the moment and use your eyes and body to engage your audience.

Pro tip

Caressing your body in this way might feel weird at first, but it's all part of the challenge that Burlesque dancers face. Remember that bent knees and fishnet tights help to create a fabulous silhouette, and anyone watching will be mesmerized by this sexy move. So don't hold back – throw away the stresses of life and frame your beautiful body.

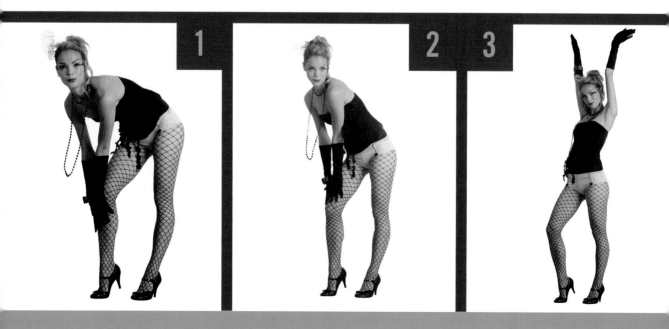

Side and front shimmy

1 Move your hands down your body so they end up at hip level. With your left leg bent and facing the left-hand corner of the room, lean forwards and shake your shoulders rapidly from side to side. This is known as a shimmy.

2 Repeat the move facing in the opposite direction and with your right leg bent.

3 Finish the movement with a shimmy straight to the front.

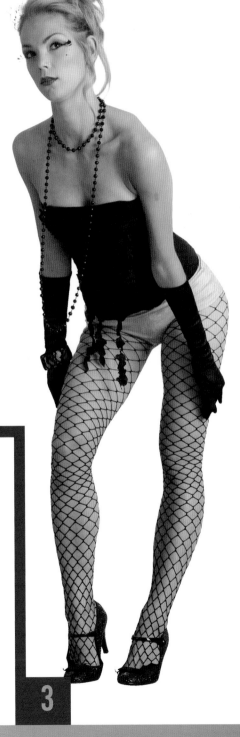

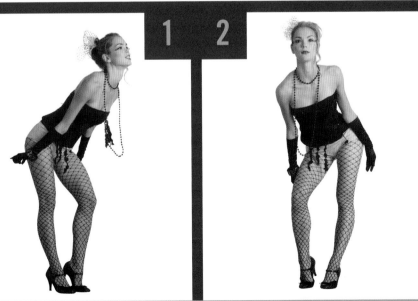

Cross-over steps with kicks

1—2 Leading with your right foot, walk four steps to the left, crossing your feet over as you go.

3 When you finish walking, cross your arms over your chest, so your right hand is resting on your left shoulder and your left hand is resting on your right shoulder. Shimmy for three seconds.

4 Leading with your left foot, walk four steps to the right – this should take you back to where you were. Cross your arms over in the same way as before and shimmy again for three seconds.

5 End the move by kicking your left foot out to the right. Don't worry about height, just lift your leg three inches off the floor and flick it seductively away in the direction that your body is facing.

Repeat the move, this time kicking your right leg to the left, following the general direction of your body. Flick your foot out and flirt with the air!

❝ Since taking up Burlesque dancing my self-esteem has gone through the roof and I feel fantastic about the future. ❞

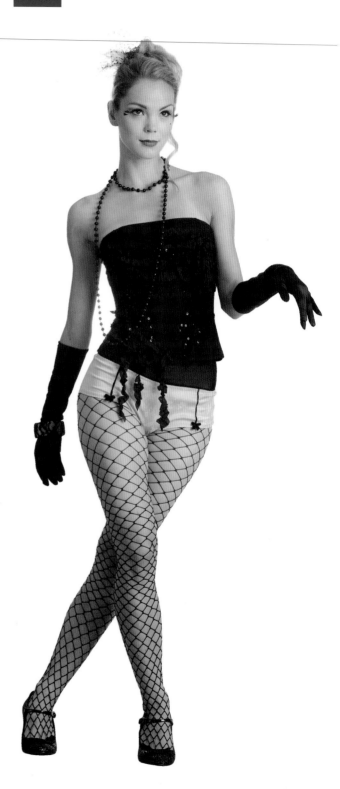

2 3

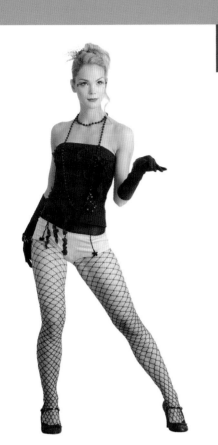

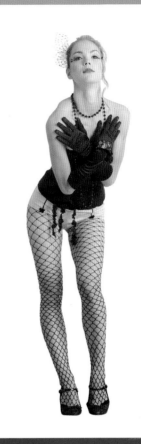

4 5

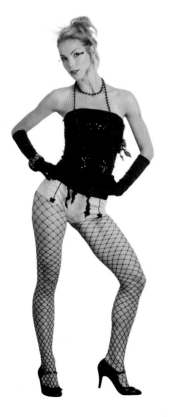

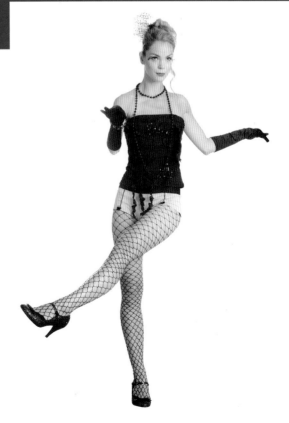

Side step walk with arms

1 Cross your left foot over your right foot and your left hand over your right hand in front of you.

2 Extend your right foot out to the side and point your toes. You won't move very far, but you'll make a great picture with your body. Use your arms and hips creatively to make a definite pose, keeping your eyes forwards at all times.

Repeat the movement, except this time cross your right foot over your left foot and extend your left foot out to the side. Pose again. Repeat this move twice more – once on the right, once on the left.

Pro tip

There's no such thing as a typical Burlesque act. Some girls play the role of femme fatale, others go for girlie and coy. Whatever approach you decide on, use the posed moments of this dance to make a statement about your showgirl character. Tease, tempt, or turn on the charm. Don't let the final moments of the dance pass by without maximising the drama and going for a stunning final pose!

1

2

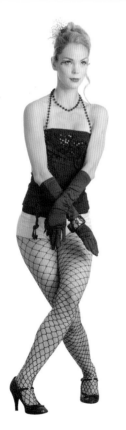

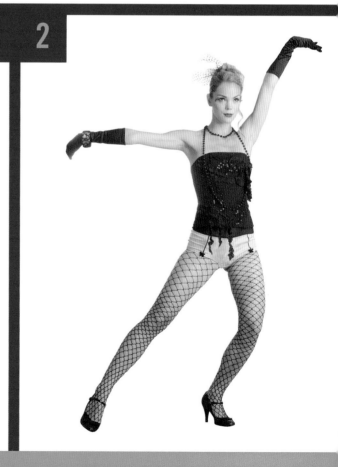

Turn and final pose

1 Spin round in a clockwise direction so you are facing the back of the room.

2 Walk four steps towards the back, circling your hands at hip level as you walk.

3 Pivot on your heels in a clockwise direction and execute a final pose. Any confident pose will work, but why not start with this idea: place your right arm on your right hip (elbow bent), and plunge your left arm into the air, behind your left ear.

Keep your fingers splayed. Bend your knees so that one hip is tilted slightly higher than the other. Look your audience in the eye and wink. Dita Von Teese – eat your heart out!

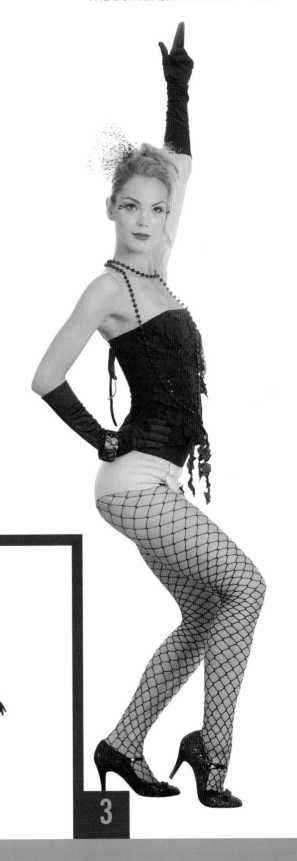

1 2

3

Burlesque dancing for your fitness level

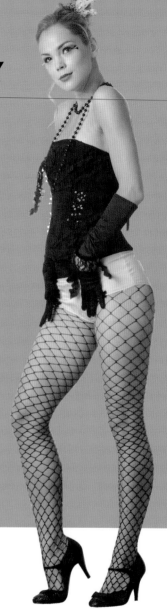

Burlesque is not the kind of dance that should be prescribed and altered according to your fitness level. It's not about repetitions or sets of movements, it's about teasing, playing and enjoying being a woman. For this reason, anyone can dance the routine, regardless of your fitness level.

However, if you want to increase the rapidity of your movements and make Burlesque an aerobic as well as creative challenge, choose a song from the Super-fit playlist and keep up to speed with the beat. If you want to keep things slow and sultry, play something from the Getting Fit playlist. And if you're happy trying something midway between the two, go for a song from Fighting Fit.

Whatever you do, remember to perform your moves with enthusiasm and commitment. You'll be stunned by the results.

Burlesque playlists

GETTING FIT
(level 1)

1. Peggy Lee
   'Fever'
2. Pussycat Dolls
   'Feelin' Good'
3. Nina Simone
   'Sugar In My Bowl'

FIGHTING FIT
(level 2)

1. Marilyn Monroe
   'Diamonds Are A Girl's Best Friend'
2. The Creed Taylor Orchestra
   'The Nervous Beat'
3. Pussycat Dolls
   'Tainted Love'

SUPER-FIT
(level 3)

1. Barney Kessell
   'Honey Rock'
2. Goldfrapp
   'Ride On A White Horse'
3. Eartha Kitt
   'Just An Old Fashioned Girl'

Case study

Claire Thrift, 28, a music features editor from London, took up Burlesque dancing in 2004 after her husband, Richard, bought her lessons for her birthday. Here she explains how showgirl dancing has toned her body and made her feel more fabulous than ever before...

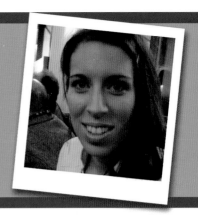

'I was really nervous on the day of my first Burlesque class, but as soon as I met my teacher, Jo King, I knew I had nothing to worry about. Jo made it clear from the start that women of all shapes and sizes can dance Burlesque. In the Burlesque scene, curves are seen as a fabulous thing, and she ordered us all to stop dieting and start flaunting our bodies. I didn't expect to hear this from a dance teacher and it put me at ease instantly.

'After just one class I realized Burlesque was working wonders for my body. I've never had a bad body image, but before I started the course I wasn't especially toned and sometimes I cringed when I caught a glimpse of myself naked. I'm tall, but my posture wasn't brilliant and often I'd walk into a crowded party and wish I was a bit shorter and less noticeable.

'However, Burlesque dancing made me feel more confident straight away. The act I developed involves lots of stretching and floor work and by the end of every class I'd feel like I'd done two hours of yoga. By the end of the course, my thighs were longer and leaner than before and my waist had slimmed

'An hour of Burlesque makes me feel like the most attractive, most fantastic woman in the world.'

down. I also became more aware of the way I carry myself, leading to an improvement in my posture. I stopped wanting to disappear when I walked into a room and starting strutting confidently thorough crowds instead!

'Five months after finishing my course, I auditioned for a regular dancing slot at a club called Volupté in London. I never imagined I'd become a professional dancer, but now I perform once a week to audiences ranging from 30 to 300 people. I've got a professional stage name – Lux Fonteyne – and after a show I come out feeling like the sexiest, most attractive, fantastic woman in

the world. It's like I'm oozing sexuality and body confidence and quite honestly, this feeling lasts. Rich has noticed that since taking up Burlesque I'm a happier person. I used to get really stressed about where my career was going, but dancing has helped to calm my inner critic and relax me.

'My tip for anyone trying Burlesque for the first time is to turn the music up loud, slip on your sexiest shoes and lock the living room door. Forget your inhibitions and give it a go. Don't skip this chapter just because you're not super-confident right now: any woman in need of an ego boost should definitely try Burlesque. After a few practice sessions, you'll swap dancing in front of your mirror for dancing in front of your man. You'll love it, and I'm sure he won't complain either!'

Index

AND counts 39
arch-ups 35
arms
　Broadway arm and leg
　　flick 68
　Burlesque arms up and
　　over the body 128-9
　Burlesque side step
　　walk with arms 138

back and front kicks 31
back problems 8
back stretches 26, 27
ballet foot positions 28,
　29, 30
ballet-style exercises 28-
　31
bangle 112-13
bare feet 15, 19
benefits of dancing see
　health and fitness
　benefits
Bhangra see Bollywood
body confidence
　developing see case
　　studies
　lack of 9
body flick 76-7
body roll 46-7, 50-1
body toning 8
　see also case studies
Bollywood 13, 98
　bangle 112-13
　case study 119
　double leg pushy pushy
　　106-7
　fitness levels 118
　forward and back step
　　102-3
　Indian bop step 101
　Indian classical hands
　　100
　jump jump heel 104-5
　kit 15
　leg drops 114-15
　shunting 110-11
　twists 108-9, 116-17
bop step, Indian 101
bottom shimmy 132-3
bounce and shake 50-1
bridging 34
Broadway 13, 59

arm and leg flick 68
body flick 76-7
building the drama 60-1
case study 79
click steps 66
fitness levels 78
Fosse style 67
kit 14
leg lift 74-5
overhead claps 62-3
pirouette 72-3
playlists 78
posing 64
side show 65
step and kick 70-1
step and turn 69
stepping back 67
travelling step 65
building the drama 60-1
bumps 124, 130
Burlesque 13, 121
　bottom shimmy 132-3
　case study 141
　cross-over steps with
　　kicks 136-7
　fitness levels 140
　framing, caressing and
　　posing 134
　grind turn 131
　grinding and front
　　bumps 130
　kit 14
　playlists 140
　pose and wiggle 122-3
　side and front shimmy
　　135
　side step walk with
　　arms 138
　side steps 126-7
　turn and final pose 139
　walk and front four-step
　　125
　wiggle and side bumps
　　124

calf stretch, standing 25
cardiovascular fitness 8
case studies
　Bollywood 119
　Broadway 79
　Burlesque 141
　Hip Hop 57
　Latin 97
　Tango 97
cat back stretch 27
Cha Cha 86-7, 89

claps, overhead 62-3
click steps 66
clothing 14-15
confidence
　developing see case
　　studies
　lack of 9
core strength exercises 32
costumes 14-15
counts
　Hip Hop 39
　Latin 82
cross-over steps with
　kicks 136-7
crunches 32

dance kit 14-15
dance style quiz 10-13
dance trainers (footwear)
　14, 15
Dent, Rebecca (Broadway
　case study) 79
destressing 8
dips, tricep 35
double leg pushy pushy
　106-7

facing the front 42-3
final pose, Hip Hop 54-5
first position, ballet 28,
　29, 30
fitness levels 8, 9, 18, 19
　Bollywood 118
　Broadway 78
　Burlesque 140
　Hip Hop 56
　Latin 96
flexibility 9
flicks
　Broadway arm and leg
　　flick 68
　Broadway body flick
　　76-7
　Latin Tango walk and
　　leg flick 94-5
foot positions, ballet 28,
　29, 30
footwear 14-15, 19
forward and back step
　102-3
forward lunges
　Hip Hop 44-5
　warm up 20
forward stretch 25
Fosse, Bob (Broadway
　choreographer) 67

four-step, front 125
framing, caressing and
　posing 134
front and back kicks 31
front bumps 130
front four-step 125
front shimmy 92-3

grind turn 131
grinding and front bumps
　130

half crunches 32
half press-ups 33
hamstring stretch,
　standing 26
hands, Indian classical
　100
head and neck stretches
　23
health and fitness
　benefits 8
　Bollywood 108
　Broadway 63
　Burlesque 126
　Hip Hop 45
　Latin 87
　see also case studies
heeled shoes 14, 15
Hip Hop 13, 37
　body roll 46-7, 50-1
　bounce and shake 50-1
　case study 57
　counts 39
　facing the front 42-3
　final pose 54-5
　fitness levels 56
　forward lunge 44-5
　kit 15
　off-lock 38
　playlists 56
　scoop move 38-9
　shoulder roll 48
　tick tock 52-3
　timing 39
　turn 49
　walking 40-1
hip opener 27
hip rolls 24
hip stretch 28
hip swing 82-3

Indian bop step 101
Indian classical hands
　100
injury prevention 18

joints 18, 29
jumps
    Bollywood jump jump
        heel 104-5
    warm up sideways
        jumps and punches
        21
    warm up star jumps 20

kicks
    Broadway step and kick
        70-1
    Burlesque cross-over
        steps with kicks
        136-7
    warm up front and
        back kicks 31
killer moves
    Bollywood 104-5
    Broadway 72-3
    Burlesque 130-1
    Hip Hop 52-3
    Latin 86-7
kit 14-15, 19
knee bends and shoulder
    circles 23
knees popping 29

Latin 13, 81
    case study 97
    counts 82
    fitness levels 96
    front shimmy 92-3
    hip swing 82-3
    kit 15
    playlists 96
    salsa steps 84-5, 88
    side-front steps and
        Cha Cha 86-7, 89
    Tango walk and leg flick
        94-5
    timing 82
    turns 90-1
leg drops 114-15
leg flicks
    Broadway arm and leg
        flick 68
    Latin Tango walk and
        leg flick 94-5
leg lift 74-5
lunges see forward lunges

Mambo 86
marching on the spot 20
mirrors 122
muscle tone 8

music see playlists

neck and head stretches
    23

off-lock 38
Olton, David (Bollywood
    choreographer) 98
overhead claps 62-3

pace see fitness levels
pain 18
performance mode 17,
    60, 138
physical capabilities see
    fitness levels
pirouettes 72-3
plank 34
playlists
    Broadway 78
    Burlesque 140
    Hip Hop 56
    Latin 96
pliés 29
    plié with stretch 22
popping knees 29
posing
    Broadway 64
    Burlesque 122-3, 134,
        138, 139
    Hip Hop 54-5
postural problems 8
press-ups 33-5
punches, sideways jumps
    and 21
pushy pushy, double leg
    106-7

quad stretch, standing 26
quiz 10-13

rises 30
rolls
    Hip Hop body roll 46-7,
        50-1
    Hip Hop shoulder roll
        48
    warm up hip rolls 24

salsa steps 84-5, 88
Schwartz, Kim (Latin
    Tango case study) 97
scoop move 38-9
second position, ballet 29,
    30
Sedani, Sejal (Bollywood

case study) 119
shake, Hip Hop bounce
    and 50-1
shimmy
    Burlesque bottom
        shimmy 132-3
    Burlesque side and
        front shimmy 135
    Latin front shimmy 92-3
shoes 14-15, 19
shoulder circles and knee
    bends 23
shoulder roll 48
shunting 110-11
side body bend 24
side bumps 124
side and front shimmy
    135
side show 65
side steps
    Burlesque side step
        walk with arms 138
    Burlesque side steps
        126-7
    Latin side-front steps
        and Cha Cha 86-7,
        89
    warm up side step and
        reach 21
sideways jumps and
    punches 21
sit ups (crunches) 32
spotting 72
stamina building 9
standing calf stretch 25
standing hamstring
    stretch 26
standing quad stretch 26
star jumps 20
step and kick 70-1
step and turn 69
stepping back 67
stilettos 14
stress 8
stretching exercises 22-8
sweeping stretch 27

Tango
    case study 97
    Tango walk and leg flick
        94-5
third position, ballet 29,
    30
Thrift, Claire (Burlesque
    case study) 141
tick tock 52-3

timing
    Hip Hop 39
    Latin 82
toe stretch 28
trainers (footwear) 14, 15,
    19
travelling step 65
tricep dips 35
turns
    Broadway step and turn
        69
    Burlesque grind turn
        131
    Burlesque turn and
        final pose 139
    Hip Hop 49
    Latin 90-1
twists, Bollywood 108-9,
    116-17
two left feet 9

walking
    Burlesque side step
        walk with arms 138
    Burlesque walk and
        front four-step 125
    Hip Hop walking 40-1
    Latin Tango walk and
        leg flick 94-5
wall press-ups 33
warm up 17, 19
    ballet-style exercises
        28-31
    core strength exercises
        32
    press-ups 33-5
    starting exercises 20-1
    stretching exercises 22-
        8
weight loss see case
    studies
wiggles, Burlesque 122-3,
    124
Wilson, Zievrina (Hip Hop
    case study) 57
worries 9

Acknowledgements

The workouts in this book have been devised by the following
dance experts:

The Warm Up: Caroline Graham – Caroline is a trained physiotherapist and
dancer from Huddersfield, west Yorkshire. In 2004 she won Channel 4's
Musicality competition and made her West End debut playing Velma Kelly in
Chicago. In 2005 she joined the UK touring cast of *Saturday Night Fever* for
12 months.

The Hip Hop Workout: Lil 'J – Lil' J teaches has been dancing since the 1980s
and has a B. Ed in Dance and Drama. For more information, see her website:
www.lil-j.co.uk

The Broadway Workout: Linda Dadd – Linda trained as a jazz dancer and has
performed in various shows, videos and commercials. For more
information, see www.pineapple.uk.com

The Latin Workout: Serena Bobowski – Serena trained in Flamenco, Salsa, and
Afro-Brazilian dance at the Centre du Danse au Marais in Paris. She now teaches
Pilates and is a founding member of the theatre collective Shunt.

The Bollywood Workout: David Olton – David trained at the Stella Mann School
of Dance (ballet) and the Laban Centre (contemporary dance). He has performed
in several West End shows, including Andrew Lloyd Webber's Bollywood musical,
Bombay Dreams. For more information on David, see www.yogaballetfusion.com

The Burlesque Workout: Jo King – Jo is founder and director of
the London School of Striptease. She has over 20 years' experience as
a professional Burlesque performer and cabaret artist. For more information
about Jo and her company, see www.londonschoolofstriptease.co.uk.

Physio advice: Jackie Pelly
Head physiotherapist, English National Ballet

Author Acknowledgements
Special thanks to Jess Spiring and Zoë Seymour at Zest for coming to me with
this exciting project, and for supporting me all the way through. Thanks also to
Victoria Alers-Hankey and Carly Madden at Collins & Brown. Sincere thanks to
David, Jo, Linda, Lil' J, Serena and Caroline for devising the fabulous workouts
for this book. Thanks also to Kim, Claire, Rebecca, Sejal and Zievrina for sharing
your inspiring stories with me. Huge thanks to Claudia Ginsburg, Rachel Branton,
Jennifer Tanarez and Gemma Pritchard for their help with various stages of the
book. And lastly – but not least – thanks to my wonderful family and friends for
putting up with my anti-social working hours and for encouraging a girl to have
her dreams! I hope you all enjoy the book.